MW00474334

The Kelee

*An Understanding of
the Psychology of Spirituality*

The Kelee

An Understanding of the Psychology of Spirituality

Ron W. Rathbun

QUIESCENCE PUBLISHING
OCEANSIDE, CALIFORNIA

THE KELEE
An Understanding of
the Psychology of Spirituality

This book is an original publication of Quiescence^SM Publishing

PRINTING HISTORY
Quiescence Publishing first edition / March 2004

For information address:
Quiescence Publishing
Post Office Box 373
Oceanside, CA 92049-0373
www.ronrathbun.com

ISBN: 0-9643519-8-6

Library of Congress Control Number: 2003098270

PRINTED IN THE UNITED STATES OF AMERICA

Acknowledgements

There are many people I would like to thank
for helping to develop the deep understanding
of the Kelee over the last two decades.

All of these individuals know who they are
and how they have helped. There are no words
to describe my appreciation, other than
a heart-felt, loving—*thank you*.

*Each day
has its own beauty,
when you are open
to accept it.*

Contents

*When you open
your mind to see,
you will.*

Preface

All masters throughout time have said one thing, "Your answers are within you." Now for the first time ever, here is a direct map to your heart. In understanding the Kelee, you will unlock the mysteries of your mind. The Kelee (pronounced "key-lee") brings together a clear relationship between psychology and spirituality. It's time for everyone to understand that the mind and spirit are not separate.

Through decades of studying what works and what does not, I found a way to free myself from my emotional pain permanently. What I found was startling: a way to understand my mind from the inside out. It really is possible to free yourself from your issues and open your mind to love life.

If you look at life in the most basic terms, you will find that everyone is looking for one thing; it's to feel good inside about one's self and the world around us. But how each individual achieves this is altogether different. To start, it's important to ask yourself, "Do I like who I am?" and "What do I want to change about myself?" If you want to change, are you trying to create a new state of mind or are you trying to clean up your existing one?

If you're trying to create a state of mind, you must ask yourself, "How can I create that which I do not understand or feel?" If you already feel a happy state of mind, why would you need to create another one? Ultimately all you can do is clean up what you already have. Nevertheless, how do you do this?

First, it's important to look at what's blocking you from feeling happiness. It's always negative compartmentalized thoughts or your issues. Do you have issues that you cannot get rid of, but say you're working on them? How are you working on them? And even if you could drop your issues, it would be like dropping a heavy backpack in the desert, with no water to drink. How you drink of life comes from opening your spirit to fulfillment, but how do you do that?

How would you like to do a practice for your mind that will make every day better? The Kelee is what distinguishes this practice from all others. The Practice in this book is formally called The Kelee Meditation Practice. Students just call it The Practice, so in this book I will refer to it as The Practice. This practice will show you how to calm brain function, dissolve your fear-based issues, and open your conscious awareness to connect with your spirit directly.

The Practice is one of the most amazing techniques for the mind you will ever experience. The Kelee is only hidden from people because without training you only know how to see with your physical eyes, not your spiritual ones. The Practice was born out of what works and what does not. It is not a theory. Do it for yourself and see. How else do you know anything except from first hand experience? I'm sure after several months of practice, you'll either say, "This is the most valuable thing I've ever done for myself," or "Before doing this, it was as if I wasn't even living." I cannot tell you how many times I have heard these statements. But alas, as the old saying goes, talk is cheap.

Here is the knowledge that will set everyone free. The simplicity of The Practice is what will unravel the complexity of your mind. If you're fearful of this knowledge, think about this. How could you possibly think that going within your own heart and being still could be wrong in any way, shape or form? The still place in your heart is where you find peace and where love is experienced. If you want to find yourself, here is a way that has worked for those select few who are aware of it. Now for the first time it's here for everyone, if you can see its beauty and truthfulness.

As you read, you'll notice that I refer to three key elements. On the following page I explain how these elements are interconnected.

Here are the three basic ways your conscious awareness operates:

1. In brain function—the two physical hemispheres of the brain associated with the intellect.

2. In mind function—the observing part of us associated with the spirit.

3. In dysfunction—compartmentalization of negative issues trapped in the Kelee.

Compartments operate in three basic ways:

1. Adrenaline compartments that explode outward.

2. Depression compartments that turn inward.

3. Self-created reality compartments that escape to a world within your mind.

The conscious awareness is affected by compartments in three ways:

1. Being consumed—when your conscious awareness is consumed by a compartment and you are unaware that you're completely controlled by it.

2. Being influenced—when your conscious awareness feels the effect of a compartment and you're aware of it but you're not controlled by it.

3. Being free—when your conscious awareness is unaffected by compartmentalization and you are totally aware of your freedom.

In reading this book you'll see a diagram on the left side of the page. It is a basic line drawing of the Kelee and shows the direction that energy flows within it. The arrows pointing to the Kelee diagram are general in nature. Depending on the topic covered the arrows will point to the brain and the lesser Kelee, the surface of the mind or the greater Kelee and the spirit.

The Practice will teach you how to know yourself. The diagram of the Kelee is a map to self-understanding. If you want to cultivate true mental strength, you will have to practice. Sit down, do The Practice and you will see for yourself, the greatest adventure of all starts within your mind. If you want to explore the unknown reaches of your mind, let the journey begin.

*When you do something good
for yourself
you do something good
for everybody.*

Chapter One

The Practice

An ancient wisdom says,
"Practice makes perfect."
It's true.

*When you relax
your conscious awareness,
tension in the mind
will reveal itself as compartments.*

Tension blocks the mind's
sensitivity to perception

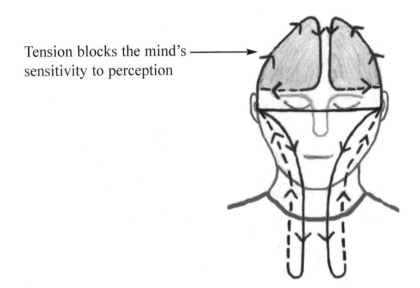

Everyone has tension and it's important for overall health to be able to let go of it. If you cannot let go of tension, you will not be able to move deeper into mind function. Relaxation should not be something that you do only occasionally. It would be wise to be relaxed daily. It's important to let go of every ounce of tension in your mind every day. Think of doing your practice as your time to be good to yourself.

When you start doing The Practice, you'll run into tension in the lesser Kelee region from compartments. **Step One** of The Practice is to feel your conscious awareness at the top of your head and then feel your conscious awareness relax and soften. When your conscious awareness is in your feeling sense, you'll notice the tension in your brain. You'll probably find a mass of tension in your brain, but over time as you continue, you'll begin to relax and sense isolated tight areas. As your conscious awareness relaxes and your sensitivity opens, you'll begin to feel blocks of tension known as compartments. Now you can start to troubleshoot your Kelee because you can *feel*; your ability to feel will develop into a sense called awareness, this is in actuality your sixth sense. With this newly developed awareness, you'll learn many things about yourself. Now you're on your way to self-awareness, which is the process of self-understanding.

This is the path to enlightenment, otherwise known simply as a way to live. When a relaxed state of mind opens your perception to self-understanding, the path to enlightenment becomes very real.

*The price you pay
for being wound up and tense
is at the expense of your ability
to wind down and relax.*

Tension in the brain hinders ⟶
access to the mind i.e., spirit

When you first start doing The Practice, one of the things you will notice is how much tension you're carrying in your head. This tension is caused by brain function, wanting to do too much, or from compartments that have their own independent tension. If you carry this much tension in your head, you will have to decompress to be able to drop into your greater Kelee. This will take patience because dissipating tension takes time. If the tension only dissolves at one or two percent a day and you need to get to fifty-one percent to recognize how tight you are, you may get frustrated and think The Practice is not working. This is extremely common for people in the early stages of The Practice. Do your practice regardless and trust that calming your mind is beneficial. Who really wants to be uncomfortable with the weakness that stress and tension bring to your mind, not to mention all of the harm it does to your immune system and body?

Tension limits access to your mind i.e., spirit. You will have no idea what this means until you begin to release built up stress through The Practice. When the shift happens and you're more relaxed than tense, I assure you, you will like it. There are no negative effects from The Practice other than having to face the compartments causing your negativity! Release your tension and you will drain your negative compartments.

Mental tension and relaxation are at two opposite ends of a spectrum. Where would you like to be?

*Without discipline
in The Practice,
there can be no follow-through.*

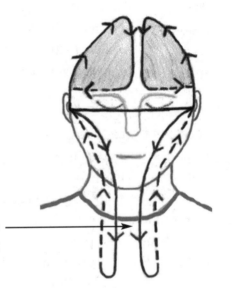

The discipline you seek is ——————
from your mind i.e., spirit

If you are going to succeed at anything, you must have discipline. If you want to experience the beautiful effects of The Practice, you must be consistent enough to see results.

The small mind of your brain will do everything in its power to not give up control to your big mind i.e., spirit. It will create a million excuses why you shouldn't give yourself five minutes in the morning and five minutes in the evening to do your practice, none of them valid. Have you ever heard the phrase, "Cleanliness is next to godliness"? You wash the outside of your body every day. How about washing what's running your body? When your Kelee is clean, you'll be clean. Ten minutes out of twenty-four hours is about one percent of your day. If you can't give yourself one percent out of your day, are you in control of your life?

As you do The Practice, you will begin to see results within a few days to a few weeks, depending on your level of awareness and discipline. At six months your progress will be distinct and at one year profound. After about a year I ask students, "How have you changed?" or "What's the difference between now and back before you started The Practice?" Invariably they will shake their head and say, "It was as if I wasn't even living before."

The Practice will be the most valuable thing you will ever do for yourself. Your development will only end when you attain full enlightenment, and who's worried about that?

*Doing The Practice
is like having a job
if you don't go to work,
you don't get paid.*

Letting go of your body, opens you to your mind

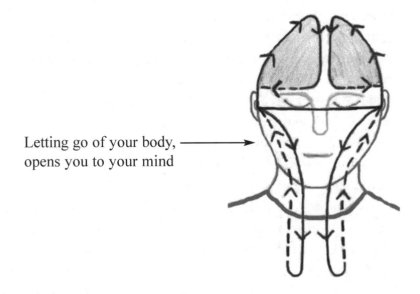

Where to do your practice. Find a quiet place in your home free from distractions. If there are others around, inform them that you're doing your practice and to not disturb you for a while. Do not associate your practice with a special place; don't make an attachment to a location. Simply find a quiet place to sit.

When to do your practice. Do your practice in the morning as early as you can, before your mind becomes too active with the day to come or it may not get done. Do your evening practice before you get too tired because if your energy level is down, it will be too easy to fall asleep. Your practice is considered successful if you did it, no matter how still your mind was in it.

How to sit in your practice. Sit in a comfortable position with your spine erect and your hands resting comfortably; this is simply good posture. It's OK to sit cross-legged or in a chair, as long as you're comfortable. If your body is uncomfortable, you will not be able to let go of it. You will be distracted while you're in the lesser Kelee and not be able to drop into the greater Kelee. Do not lie down to do your practice; it's too easy to go to sleep. You must teach your mind how to relax without going to sleep. You already know how to sleep, but you don't know how to still your mind, yet.

Props and The Practice. You don't need any! Anything that is used as a prop will end up being a psychological crutch. The purest state of mind is found through the mind itself.

The Practice will dissolve all dysfunction with practice, persistence and patience.

*The Practice starts
with your physical eyes closed
and your mind open.*

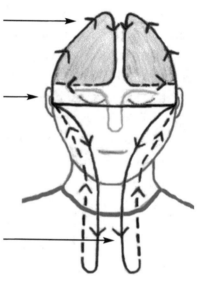

Step One of The Practice
starts at the top of your head
and relaxes down through
both hemipheres of the brain
to the surface of the mind,
for about 2 minutes

While at the surface of the
mind, relax across it for
about 30 seconds

Step Two begins when you
drop into your greater Kelee.
The second step ends after
about 3 minutes

Step Three occurs upon
returning to the surface of the
mind, take another 5 minutes
for introspection and
contemplation

In **Step One** of The Practice, *you have a relaxed awareness of self, but you are not thinking.* This is extremely important! The Practice is about allowing your conscious awareness to get still, not forcing it to. The reason for spreading out your conscious awareness and relaxing it across the surface of your mind is that there are always compartments stored there that need to be dissolved.

Step Two of The Practice is about totally letting go of sense consciousness, and allowing your conscious awareness to drop to a point in your greater Kelee, where you remain as still as you can for about three minutes. While you're in the first two steps of The Practice you'll be tempted to watch what's going on in your Kelee. If you do, you'll start thinking this is not The Practice but you in a normal waking state of thinking. To continue your growth, remember that The Practice is about stilling your mind, not thinking!

Step Three is when you come back to the surface of your mind to full awareness and begin the process of introspection and contemplation. Do not hurry into your day!

The Practice is a priceless gift you can give to yourself. You receive from it by doing it.

When the brain is not thinking,
the mind can begin quieting.

Step One of The Practice ⟶
begins at the top of your
head with your eyes closed

And proceeds down to the ⟶
surface of the mind

The Practice starts by bringing your conscious awareness to the top of your head using your feeling process. The feeling process is associated with your spirit i.e., mind function. If you're having a hard time feeling your conscious awareness at the top of your head, try this: touch the tips of your fingers together and you'll notice you can feel them. Now with your finger tips, touch the top of your head and you'll feel your awareness there. *It is extremely important that you pay attention to this point!* It will take some practice but you will improve.

In **Step One** bring your conscious awareness to the top of your head by using thought command, this will direct your conscious awareness from mind function. When you've been operating mostly from the brain i.e., intellect, it will take some time to shift into mind function on command. If you cannot get into the feeling process of mind function, your conscious awareness will be absorbed into the thinking process of the brain or compartments as you pass through them, while in the lesser Kelee. When doing **Step One** of The Practice you can actually feel an awareness of self as you move slowly down through both hemispheres of the brain and not be actively thinking. Remember, the entire practice is about not thinking.

This first step of The Practice will begin moving your conscious awareness into mind function, and at the same time begin dissolving compartments in the lesser Kelee. All it takes is practice, persistence and patience.

*The brain operates
in three dimensions,
but it takes the mind
to understand them.*

The brain operates in
planes of awareness

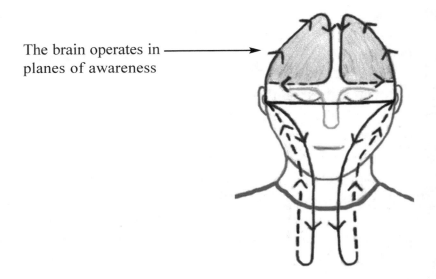

The brain and our physical self operate in a three-dimensional world of height, width and depth. The brain is comfortable with planes of awareness associated with a linear state of thinking because that's how it relates with the world.

In **Step One** of The Practice, feel your conscious awareness at the top of your head, make sure that your conscious awareness is moving down as a horizontal plane of awareness through both hemispheres of your brain. You are not visualizing this plane; you are feeling a relaxed awareness of self. It is extremely important that you understand this point from the start. As this plane of awareness relaxes and softens, your conscious awareness shifts into mind function, dissolving compartments while passing through them.

The energy of the lesser Kelee is three-dimensional in how it folds in and around both hemispheres of the brain. As you do The Practice in the lesser Kelee area, you'll experience times when your plane of awareness tilts and it's difficult to move through both hemispheres of your brain. What you're running into is electrochemical resistance from compartments. Relax and soften your awareness even more, and you'll effortlessly pass though the resistance. It may seem like you're doing nothing, but be assured, you're doing something.

It will take some time before you realize that the energy of your spirit initially appears as nothing significant, but in actuality carries the greatest significance of all.

*Relaxation is not a creation
or a visualization of energy,
it's allowing yourself
to be relaxed.*

A relaxed awareness of self
is how you start The Practice

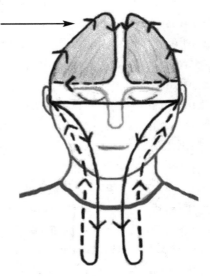

It is common for people when doing **Step One** of The Practice—from the top of the head down to the surface of the mind—to visualize and project their awareness from the surface of their mind up to the top of their head.

Do not do this! If you visualize, it will keep you in brain function and split your conscious awareness between two points at the same time. You do not want to split your conscious awareness. What you're trying to do is shift the balance of power from the small mind i.e., brain function, to the big mind i.e., mind function. You're trying to move into mind function and detach from brain function. In reality, what you're trying to do is clean up the condition of your mind, you're not trying to visualize or create a new state of mind. Visualization is great for doing some things in the world but it doesn't help you understand yourself. Understanding yourself is about knowing the true nature of your mind.

When you do The Practice and if you're a visual person, watch if your conscious awareness is connected to your physical eyes. If you cannot let go of sense consciousness associated with your physical eyes, it will be difficult to let go of brain function. You'll know you're in brain function if your eyes move upward when you go to the top of your head. When you have moved into mind function, your eyes will be closed and relaxed at eye level with no movement.

Shifting your awareness from brain function into mind function is the beginning of opening your mind's ability to see, otherwise known as clairvoyance.

*The Practice isn't about
how long you do it,
it's about the quality
of how you are in it.*

2 minutes from the top of
your head to the surface
of the mind

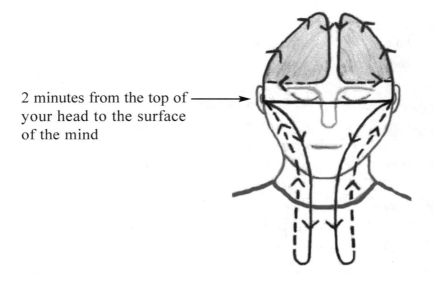

Initially people often ask, "Why is The Practice so short in duration?" The length of time to do The Practice seems short, but if you consider it would be wise to do it twice a day for the rest of your life, it isn't! *The Practice is all about the quality of stillness, not the length of time.*

Giving yourself more time to do **Step One** will not speed up how you process out compartments. The brain is fearful and tends to be stubborn; it does not like to look stupid. The brain does not like rapid change but will accept slow change. The lesser Kelee area tends to be filled with self-created comfort zone compartments that do not want to change. Everyone knows what comfort zones are—areas of your mind that are resistant to change or what is commonly called, "being set in your ways," or another way of saying, "being set in your compartments."

When you're doing **Step One** of The Practice correctly— moving slowly for about two minutes from the top of your head down to the surface of your mind—it may seem like a long time at first, but remember you do not want to be paying attention to time here, or you'll start thinking. All you do is instruct your conscious awareness to move from the top of your head down to the surface of your mind for about two minutes and it will happen. *You simply have a relaxed awareness of self without thinking.*

Be patient with The Practice and you will be most pleased.

The surface of your mind
is a worktable
where the realization
of your thought process occurs.

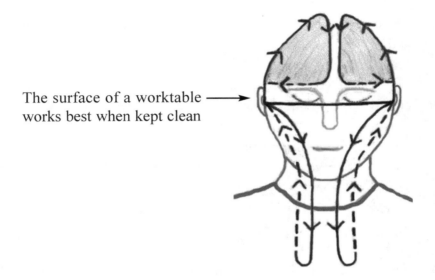

The surface of a worktable ⟶
works best when kept clean

The surface of the mind is a reception point, a point of contemplation and a place to make decisions. It would be wise to have this area easy to work from and clean.

In the last part of **Step One**—after you have come down from the top of your head to the surface of your mind—it's good to make sure your conscious awareness spreads out and softens across the entire surface of your mind. The surface of the mind has a front, sides and a back. Especially don't forget to spread your awareness to the back of your mind; people tend to keep lots of clutter there! Take about thirty seconds on this part of The Practice to feel your awareness soften, so that you can totally let go of any remaining tension from compartments before allowing yourself to drop into your greater Kelee.

It's extremely important that the surface of your mind is kept clean if you are to be comfortable with yourself and the world around you. As you start getting rid of the clutter that's collected on the surface of your mind, you'll notice how much better it feels to move around without obstacles in your way.

You can walk away from what you do in the outside world, but you can't walk away from what's on your mind. How often do you carry things on your mind? Do you like it? How would you like to not have things on your mind all of the time? When things aren't on your mind, they don't weigh on your mind.

Only you can decide how much a free mind is worth to you.

*The mind operates
in a non-linear space,
otherwise known as your spirit.*

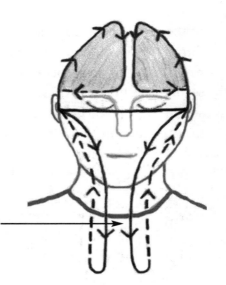

Our spirit is a state of mind
in the literal sense

Step Two of The Practice is allowing your conscious awareness to drop into your greater Kelee from the surface of your mind. If you cannot let go of tension in your brain and from compartments, you will not drop into your greater Kelee. Do not be alarmed if you have difficulty letting go in the beginning, it's common for some people to take longer to drop than others.

As you practice and relax your conscious awareness, you will drop into your greater Kelee where you will come to a natural resting point. At this resting point remain as still as you can for about three minutes without thinking. If you start to think while you're in your greater Kelee, you'll find your conscious awareness back at the surface of your mind, where thinking takes place. The object is to allow as much of your awareness down in your greater Kelee as possible, away from brain function and into mind function. This will take time because with each individual there are variables that will have a direct bearing on how controlled you are by brain function and compartmentalization. Such as, how easy or difficult your life has been.

Everything negative takes a toll on us as human beings whether we're aware of it or not. However, our saving grace is that it can all be undone through The Practice.

How everything is understood is by understanding: *What you see, is preceded by what you see.*

*A spiritual intensive
is an oxymoron
for accelerated patience.*

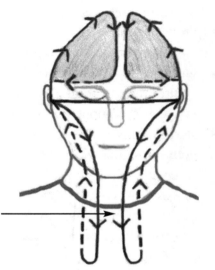

The point of living is to grow
and from a still point is how
you do it

The process of getting to a complete still point in the greater Kelee will take a long time. It's a progression and evolution that will never bottom out because there isn't one in the Kelee. There is a linear beginning when you drop from the surface of the mind, but there is no ending in the greater Kelee—it goes to infinity. The greater Kelee is a non-physical realm, where there is no matter or time—only a state of mind.

It will take a while to let go of the chatter in the brain and the compartments that have a grip on you. Nevertheless, as you relax and let go, you will move into the space that is your greater Kelee. You'll notice that when you drop from the surface of your mind down inside your greater Kelee, your conscious awareness will naturally settle to a point. This is because the mind i.e., spirit, is a point of perception. When someone asks you, "What's the point of life?"—this is it! It is from this point of perception where all life is perceived. As you continue to practice, this point will become more and more still as preconceived thoughts are dissolved and you open to the eternal moment of the now.

Your greater Kelee will open you to everything you can dream of and more. However, to open and develop your spiritual sight, you must put in the recommended three minutes in **Step Two** of The Practice. While in **Step Two** it's the quality of your stillness that's important, not the amount of time spent in your Kelee.

You cannot accelerate patience and there is no way to accelerate the moment or what you experience. There is only knowing what you experience, when you do.

*Energy without awareness
is energy
without direction.*

The brain operates in a
linear electrochemical
energy

The mind operates in a
non-linear subtle energy

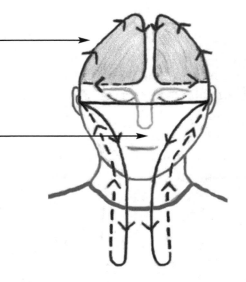

In its most basic form, the mind can only do two things: be in motion or be still. When it's in motion, what's driving the motion? Invariably it's the brain seeking sense consciousness gratification or compartments controlling behavior. These distractions make it impossible to still your mind. If your mind has no distractions—which is the spiritual law of mindfulness—it's naturally much easier to become still.

When you begin doing The Practice, you'll start to learn how much you don't understand about your energy level. You will learn how to use your energy wisely. Moderating the amount of energy you use in your brain opens your conscious awareness to your mind i.e., spirit. As you gain access to mind function, it becomes easier to deal with brain function and the dysfunction from compartments.

When you're stilling your mind, what you're trying to do is move your conscious awareness from the electrochemical energy of the brain to the subtle energy of mind in your spirit. Remember, when you're doing your practice, don't push; allow your mind to get still. A still mind is never forced; it's a natural form of stillness.

When your conscious awareness is not distracted and is at one point, stillness occurs effortlessly. This point in your waking state is where awareness, realization and understanding happen. Find this point of perception, and it will lead you out of the confusion of life. A clear point of perception is your mind's compass.

How your mind
attains stillness
is not what you think.

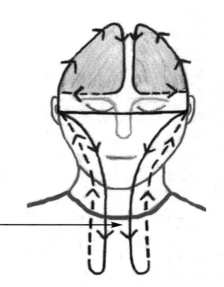

The point of stillness is to
attain nothing, which opens
you to everything

When it comes to stilling your mind, it can be a nebulous experience. So why won't your mind get still? There are several reasons:

1. The brain will not stop chattering because it's always looking to do something.

2. Compartments that seem to have a mind of their own and won't stop distracting you.

3. Your conscious awareness is thinking about all of these distractions.

As you begin doing The Practice and move more of your conscious awareness into mind function and out of brain function, you'll experience less chatter. As your conscious awareness drops into your greater Kelee, away from the surface of your mind, the remaining chatter is left behind. The longer you do The Practice and as compartments dissolve, the less distracted you will be by thoughts. As your conscious awareness attains onepointedness in your greater Kelee, you will begin to get still. Over time, this still point will develop into deeper and deeper states of awareness that in your waking state will open the spiritual eyes of your soul.

Stilling your mind is the most important and hardest thing you can do with your mind. Stillness is, in fact, what keeps your mind growing and open to change. However, you do not learn while in your practice, you learn from it after. It is extremely important to not drift off while doing The Practice or you will start thinking. It's fine to think at any other time, except while in your practice. Most importantly, your practice is about attaining stillness, not thinking about it.

Honesty
is the only policy
when it comes to true self-assessment.

Self-assessment is your
own learning curve in
your own mind

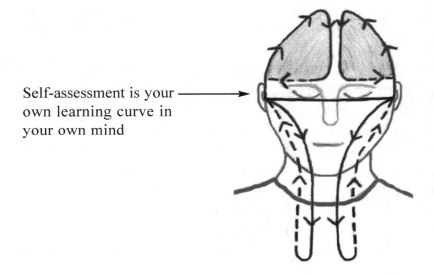

When you're doing The Practice and your mind simply will not get still, see it as such. Everything is the way it is. When you're assessing your practice and your life, be honest with yourself. Everything about doing The Practice is based on being honest with what you experience, no matter what!

When it comes to being honest with yourself, it is pass or fail: either you are honest with yourself or you are not. Do you give yourself more credit than is due, or do you not give yourself enough credit? How about acknowledging credit where credit is due? If you're not truthful with yourself, who's kidding who?

If you are driven to be right, you may want to be right at the expense of being honest with yourself. The energy behind needing to be right at any cost is ego, and always ends up as difficulty in the making, for all concerned. If you can see life truthfully, it will help you; if you cannot, it will hinder you. *You help yourself by not being other than yourself.* It's as simple as that!

When it comes to dishonesty and the mind, you get away with nothing! You can be dishonest or you can be real. Guess which way is the right way to go? Start with being honest with how you do your practice and honesty will follow you through your life.

Remember when you grade yourself too harshly; it's hard to give yourself a good grade.

The grade you give yourself,
is not nearly as important
as being honest
about the grade.

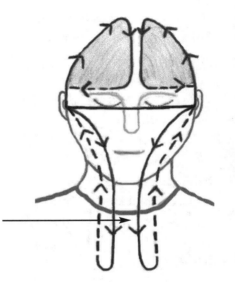

The perfect grade in The ——
Practice is a still conscious
awareness

When it comes to grading their practice, people tend to grade differently. If you start doing your practice with an ego, you will probably give yourself a better grade than you deserve. If you're shy, you'll probably give yourself less than you deserve. The goal is to be honest with yourself. If you have an active practice, grade it as such.

It will take some time to quiet the chatter of the brain and dissolve compartments. Your brain is not going to give up control easily; it's been running unchecked for your whole life. Also, your compartments are not going to give up and go away on their own. You will have to shift the balance of power, out of the dysfunction of compartments into your mind i.e., spirit, to gain control. This is why you do not want to evaluate your practice too harshly in the beginning. You're also learning patience.

Remember, assessing your practice is not to be done while in The Practice, only after. This point is extremely important; *you are not to be evaluating your practice while in it!* If you grade during your practice you will be thinking, not still. The quality of your stillness will get better. Do not give up. You have a passing grade as long as you keep trying. Your success is determined by your own efforts to help yourself. You can do this!

If you did your practice to the best of your ability, it's a success! There is no failing grade if you did your practice. You can't fail if you did it! Even if your mind would not shut up, the fact that you sat down and relaxed your mind will help you in the long term. Keep practicing!

When you detach
from what isn't you,
you find what is.

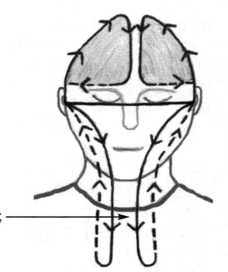

Your spirit is non-physical;
it lives in a detached world

When you learn to detach from what isn't you, you find who you really are. Who you are ultimately, is your mind i.e., spirit. Who you are not, is the negativity from compartments mistakenly taken inside as you.

Without the ability to detach from compartments, you will be forced to block out fearful feelings with your conscious awareness. When you block out negative thoughts or feelings with fear-based walls, you are inadvertently feeding your compartments. Fear feeds fear. These walls also block you from reaching your spirit, which locks you in destitution and out of the abundance of your spirit. Detachment can happen in a few ways in The Practice:

1. By moving your relaxed conscious awareness through compartments in the brain, you will dissolve them over time in the lesser Kelee. Relaxed energy is like water washing away dirt.

2. By stilling your conscious awareness to a zero point of thought—independent of compartments—you will stop feeding them with energy.

3. By living with your conscious awareness in mind function in the greater Kelee—you will detach from compartments.

These three ways of detachment will happen naturally from doing The Practice. Remember, detachment is not separation. Detachment is a feeling of connection. Separation is a feeling of disconnection.

When you're detached from what isn't you, you'll find what is you.

*Processing
is the beginning of the end
of bad moods.*

Processing is a compartment
consuming its own dysfunction

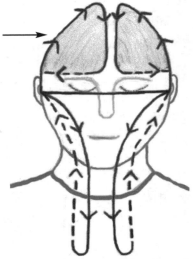

Everyone in the human equation of life runs on energy. It's just a question of what kind—negative energy from compartments or harmonious energy from your spirit. Negative energy is misperception of life; harmonious energy is clear perception of life.

When you start doing The Practice on a regular basis and begin to drop your walls that feed your compartments, you'll begin to process them out of existence. When this starts to happen, your compartments don't like it. When compartments aren't being fed energy by your conscious awareness, they begin to consume their own energy. Processing is like putting your compartments on a diet. What used to be the endless cycle of moodiness will become temporary in the form of processing.

If you've never felt compartments disappear, you will not think that you can really get rid of them. When a compartment processes out of your Kelee, you will never experience it again. This is hard to believe, but true. Issues can totally disappear from your mind through The Practice.

If you're doing The Practice correctly, the term "processing" will become a part of your vocabulary. It's much better to have the temporary effects of processing, instead of the relentless cycle of dysfunction and moodiness. Your reward for processing out a compartment is what fills in its space, your true nature, i.e., spirit. This experience can be naturally euphoric; it feels like you are being absorbed into paradise.

Processing starts the end of dysfunction and the beginning of a beautiful life experience.

*Your Kelee
is only as light or dark
as you see yourself.*

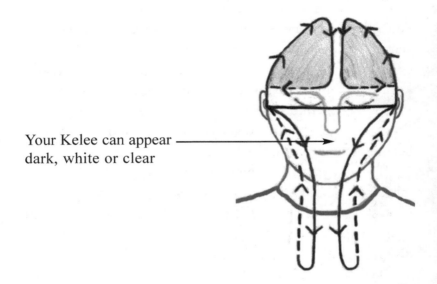

Your Kelee can appear
dark, white or clear

As you settle down with The Practice, your spiritual eyes open and you will begin to see in your Kelee. This is how it can appear:

A **dark Kelee** is when you're in the dark about yourself, making it hard to see. This darkness is because you have not consciously explored your Kelee. The darkness does not carry a negative connotation—any more than darkness at nighttime does. You're simply living in the dark about yourself. As you grow comfortable with The Practice and begin dissolving compartments, you will be less distracted and start understanding your thought process as your Kelee brightens.

A **white Kelee** is when you create reality. It appears as a mass of white energy. This white color is because you're seeing what you want to see, not what's really there. This white space can also appear as fog, which is appropriate because that's what you end up living through—a fog. This fog will eventually clear through The Practice.

A **clear Kelee** is when you are clear inside, allowing you to perceive with clarity. Clarity is the ultimate state in your Kelee. You literally are unobstructed in your thinking process. Clarity in the Kelee denotes how you perceive yourself and is the clear space everyone wants to find.

As you do The Practice and open your spiritual eyes, you'll see as you've never seen before and I assure you, you will like this state of mind!

The Kelee represents how dark, foggy or clear we experience our life. Would it not be wise to know what you can and cannot see in your mind?

All understanding starts as simple,
becomes complex
and ends back at simple.

Brain function i.e., the intellect ⟶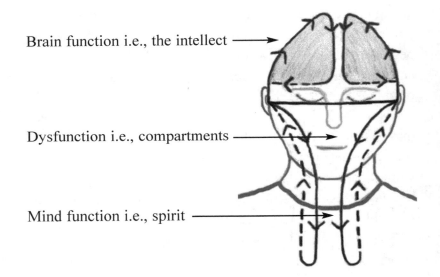

Dysfunction i.e., compartments ⟶

Mind function i.e., spirit ⟶

When you pay attention to these three parts of yourself, you will begin to understand your mind in a simple way. When your conscious awareness shifts from brain function into mind function and out of the dysfunction from compartments, your life will simply and miraculously change. When you free yourself from the dysfunction of compartments, it will feel like a miracle. Something unimaginable has changed in your soul, and you'll know it with every fiber of your being.

The simplicity of The Practice will bring about your freedom. Freedom is a space in your mind that is never controlled. Whenever we as humans are controlled, we resent it. If the feeling of being controlled is coming from your brain, you will resent it. If the feeling of being controlled is coming from your compartments, you will resent that too. Any time your mind i.e., spirit, feels controlled from outside itself, you feel imprisoned. We as humans cannot flourish in a state of mental imprisonment. It is said that the ultimate form of control is to not control at all and it's true. You're never happy when you're controlled.

Freedom in the mind leads to self-acceptance and self-acceptance leads to happiness. The Practice will shine a light on your unhappiness, dispel your confusion and open you to the simplicity of clear perception.

When you truly understand your mind, it's simple; when you don't, it's complex. Do the simple steps each day and you will see for yourself.

When you calm
the energy of your soul,
you become harmonious
with the vibration of your spirit.

The electrochemical energy of your ⟶
soul is called a beat frequency

The universal energy of your spirit ⟶
is called a baseline vibration

It seems appropriate to bring clarity to the difference between our soul and spirit. Society uses them interchangeably, but there is a difference. Your soul is who you are right now with your physical body, your conscious awareness and individual name. Your soul has an electrochemical energy called a beat frequency associated with your physical body, which is always moving up and down from food energy. The vibration from our beat frequency is one of two energies that shape us as human beings.

The second form of energy is from your spirit and is the non-physical part of you. The energy of your spirit is called a baseline vibration and is a deeper, more stable form of energy. Contained in the baseline vibration is everything known about you. It would be wise on your part to explore the energy of this vibration, which is centered in your greater Kelee.

Right now, your beat frequency is running over your baseline vibration. The closer these two sine waves are together, the more in harmony you will be. When you drop your conscious awareness into your greater Kelee, you bring these two sine waves closer together. This balances your physical and spiritual nature to oneness.

As you evolve spiritually, your name becomes less important and your spirit more important. When your physical body dies, your memories of this life will merge with your spirit, and you will move on into the spirit realm. We go somewhere, you know, and the adventure continues.

*A strong mind
is open
to what it doesn't know;
a weak mind
is open only
to what it does know.*

Chapter Two

The Basics

*The harmony
that gives you your freedom
is only determined
by your openness
to experience it.*

*There is nothing that can replace
what your own mind
can give to you.*

Your brain records intellectually
how you should live

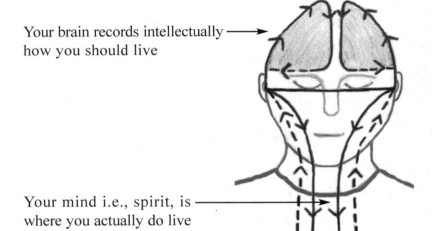

Your mind i.e., spirit, is
where you actually do live

In life, there is learning to help others and then there is learning to help yourself. How many times have you wanted to help yourself and said, "I know that intellectually but I still cannot change." Why not? If you try to change something about your mind and mentally have to keep convincing yourself you've changed, did you really change?

The brain thinks how it should live, but it doesn't feel it. If you don't know how you feel, are you living?

To first be able to help yourself, you must understand the bigger picture of collectively what our society calls mind. It seems mind can be called almost anything and yet it is something quite specific. To really understand yourself, you must understand the difference between brain function, mind function, compartments, your conscious awareness and the greater and lesser Kelee, to start. If you don't understand your mind, how can you understand your life?

If you're dysfunctional, what's the quality of how you live and what you pass on to others?

If you don't know how to actually change the condition of your mind, what do you do?

The best help you can give yourself is the understanding of how to be open with your mind.

What can be in your own mind, other than what it receives directly?

Without an open mind, you're open to nothing.

*No one can exercise
your right
to use your mind,
except you!*

Learning can be blocked by
misperception from fear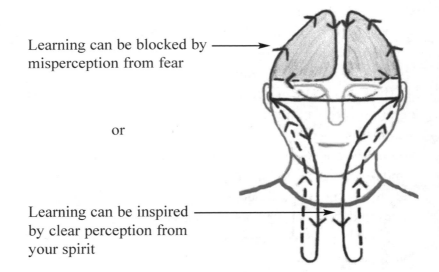

or

Learning can be inspired
by clear perception from
your spirit

There are two ways to learn: easily when inspired or difficult when fearful. Inspiring people open us up; fearful people close us down.

If you look around the world, there's lots of struggle with the learning process. The reason for difficulty with learning is due to fear-based blocks i.e., compartments sending negative messages before you start to learn. This fear can spark another big fear, looking stupid in front of others. However, what if the knowledge is required by society? Then you are forced to learn, and amazingly enough, you most often do. Nevertheless, does learning have to be forced? How much better would it be if mental blocks weren't there?

There are two basic kinds of blocks: intellectual in the lesser Kelee—in regard to doing, and spiritual in the greater Kelee—in regard to being. As you do The Practice, you will be able to dissolve all mental blocks in both areas over time. If you doubt this, unbelievably, you will learn one way or another—it's just a question of how long it will take. It's up to you how long you struggle with the learning process, whether it be intellectual or spiritual.

Learning is the process that makes us feel alive and want to explore life. Remember, if you put yourself down, who can bring you up? Open your mind to life and life will open to you.

*If you do not understand
your own thoughts,
you are spiritually illiterate.*

Intellectual literacy comes
from the brain

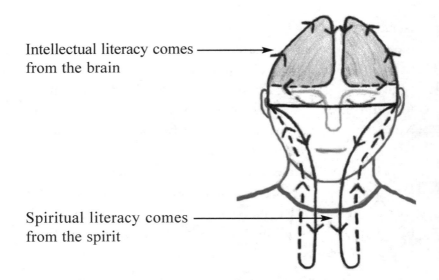

Spiritual literacy comes
from the spirit

It is a wonderful thing to be literate with the human language, but what about what the language means? This is spiritual literacy! If you are to understand your life, you must understand your thoughts.

Where do your thoughts originate?

Why is there a difference between how you think and how you feel?

When you watch a thought cross your mind, what are you watching? And if you didn't consciously think it, where did it come from?

Thoughts can come from brain function, mind function or dysfunction i.e., compartments. Unbelievably, compartments can think in place of you, with an apparent mind of their own. Scarier than that, you can actually act on what they say, without knowing where the thoughts originated. If compartments are stronger than your conscious awareness, they control you. Compartments are spiritually illiterate to wisdom and do not know what they do. Compartments do not make sense of anything; they're mindless! You can't make sense from non-sense.

As your conscious awareness learns detachment, you will begin to understand what thoughts are coming from where. If you don't have clarity in your mind, you have confusion. When you understand what the true nature of mind is—your spirit—spiritual literacy will replace confusion.

*Doing without an awareness of being
is like living
without a sense of feeling.*

The brain has a doing nature ⟶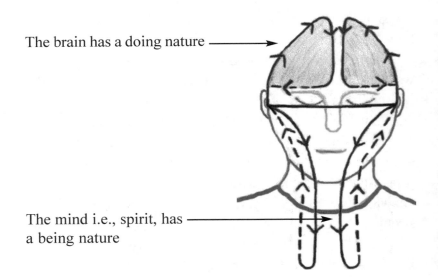

The mind i.e., spirit, has ⟶
a being nature

Doing and Being

We as humans are a dual creature, physical with a doing nature and spiritual with a being nature. This doing and being nature together brings about the complete human experience when we're in harmony.

A commonly asked question is, "How do you know the difference between brain and mind?" First, does your brain ever chatter and do you ever wish it would shut up? The chatter is coming from brain function with mind function being the observer of the chatter.

Everyone has a brain and a mind. This is part of a basic understanding of how you operate. The brain runs the memory system—the mechanics of how the physical body moves—but it's your mind i.e., spirit, that decides where and when you move. The brain instructs the body, the mind instructs the brain. If the brain operates from a doing nature without the feeling process of the spirit, your life feels devoid. If you want to have a fulfilling experience while doing, you must *feel* what you're doing. Doing without feeling our being is a mere existence; it's living outside of life. There is a reason why we are called spiritual beings.

If you really want to live, feel from your heart first, and "do" second. Remember, if you put yourself second, what you give to the world is seconds. Put your heart first and no one will ever be second.

*Sensitivity
is the mind's opening
to a deeper form of awareness.*

Sensitivity is your mind's
ability to perceive the
vibration of pain or joy

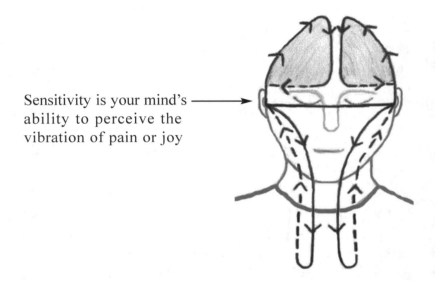

If you have pain from compartments in your mind, you may not want to look at them. If you block your pain, you desensitize your conscious awareness. If you're not sensitive, what are you, insensitive? Being closed off and cold doesn't solve anything, it only makes you cold! Who wants to be like that?

Sensitivity is not only about feeling pain, but also about the process of feeling love. It is true, *dysfunction always demands attention,* and you must deal with it, but it does not have to rule you. As you do The Practice, you set into motion your mind's ability to release yourself from the pain of misperception. Remember, all emotional pain is misperception and a block to sensitivity. The most important thing to continue your growth is your ability to still your mind. The Practice is about stilling your mind, not thinking about stilling it! Right now, you can have no idea how far The Practice will take your mind. However, if you do The Practice, you will find out.

There are levels upon levels of awareness you will perceive over time that are difficult to talk about but can be understood with great clarity. Your ability to understand the world depends on your mind's sensitivity to perceive and understand it. Sensitivity is the opening to awareness, and awareness is the opening to perceive vibrations. It's easy to hear someone's words, but can you read the vibration of what their words really mean? This takes sensitivity from a mind that has been developed.

What you are looking for in life is your own aware mind and it all starts with sensitivity!

You think what you don't know,
but you feel what you do.

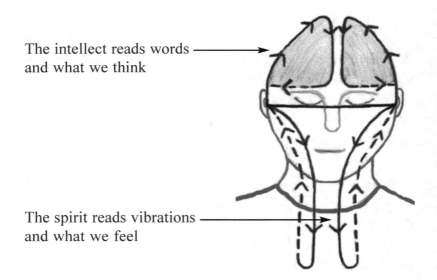

The intellect reads words
and what we think

The spirit reads vibrations
and what we feel

Whenever we meet someone, if we are somewhat aware, we get what we call a basic vibe about him or her. This vibration is a collective of this person's life experience. If they have had more experiences that are harmonious, they will be more loving. If they have had more experiences that are disharmonious, then they will be more negative. Within these two vibratory rates is every combination of human experience possible.

Quite often, it is a quandary for people to decide: do you believe what you think about someone or what you actually feel about them? If you are to develop your mind i.e., spirit, it is important to begin to trust what you sense. How many times have you had a bad feeling about something, not listened and regretted it? Have you ever noticed that if you say that you think your life is good, you are questioning it? If you feel your life is good, you do not have go up to your intellect to check. When it comes to the very deepest part of who we are, it comes down to a feeling. This deep feeling sense is associated with your spirit.

If you are to understand vibrations, you must understand mind function associated with your spirit. When you learn to read vibrations, you will never be deceived again. Vibrations can only be what they are, just as you can be only who you are. Clear your vibration with The Practice and you will open your spiritual eyes to see.

*When you understand
how you see,
seeing becomes much clearer.*

Brain function i.e., the intellect,
sees through hindsight

Dysfunction i.e., compartments,
has no sight

Mind function i.e., spirit,
sees through foresight

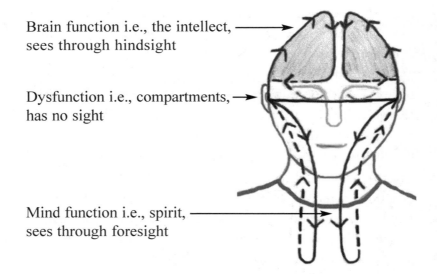

You see in three basic ways:

Brain function operates through hindsight and is one way you see life. Brain function learns through hindsight and is a memory process associated with the past. The old adage that hindsight is 20/20 is correct. The brain is helpful with performing necessary tasks in the outside world but is considered the small mind because it lacks the wisdom of mind function i.e., your spirit. Brain function operates through physical eyesight and is a linear way of thinking.

Mind function through foresight is another way you see. It is the most important ability to cultivate. Mind function involves being able to see the present clearly. You can, with training, be taught to see the potential future. Mind function operates through spiritual sight from your spirit and is a non-linear way of being.

Mind function is a feeling process that in the beginning stages of development starts as a gut level feeling and evolves into higher states of mind. Mind function is where understanding and wisdom are realized through experience.

Dysfunction from compartments is how we don't see. Compartments are mindless and cannot see at all! They can appear to have a mind of their own but in fact are mindless. They survive from what they can pull from your electrochemical energy. Dysfunction from compartments are not to be trusted, they are misperceptions of life.

*Everything
that touches your mind
influences you,
in one way or another.*

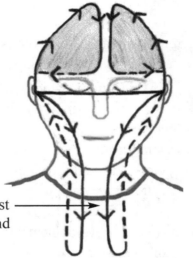

To understand yourself, you must
know what influences your mind

Virtually everyone you come in contact with will have an influence on your mind, one way or another. Every thought that passes through your mind has an influence on you, one way or another. Really think about this! It would be wise to know what influences you.

A good influence in life is always a blessing, while a negative influence feels like a curse. There's never a need to worry about good influences in the world, only the negative ones. A wise man once said, "Walk with the lame and you will learn to limp." Whom you associate with does affect you! You can always walk away from the negative influences in the outside world, but you take with you your negative compartments everywhere you go.

As you do The Practice your mind's negative influence cleans up. As you become a good influence, you will not want to hang out with negative influences. You naturally will want to live within your own mind, which, by the way, is the only place you can live anyway. You learn to be respectful of others' space. You learn that if you don't have something good to say, to not say anything. If you can't control what you say, it's a compartment talking, not you!

Why would you want to be a negative influence in the world?

The Practice is an understanding of influences, the darkness of ignorance i.e., a bad influence, and the light of awareness i.e., a good influence. A good influence comes about by cleaning up your own mind. Remember, you learn from your mind by spending time alone with it.

As wonderful as parents can be,
they cannot give
what they don't have.

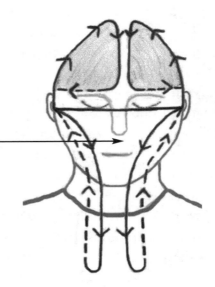

Our parents' compartments
often become our own in
the Kelee

Being a parent is the most important job on the planet, and it's sad that it takes no training whatsoever. It has long been known that issues i.e., compartments, are passed from parent to child and can be observed through generations. Just look closely at your own family. The beautiful qualities our parents pass never cause problems. However, if we do not have the spiritual puzzle pieces to protect us, their issues can become ours. It's not our parents' fault, it's what we came here to learn, and they simply provide us with an opportunity to experience what we need to grow.

Invariably, our parents, as hard as they may try not to, will probably install the biggest compartment of your life. The reason this happens is simple, when you're born, you do not have a developed mind to think for yourself. In essence, when your parents teach you, they are almost thinking for you to keep you from harming yourself. Their influence ends up in your greater Kelee as a spire of energy that your conscious awareness may default to for the rest of your life. Their influence is in between you and the true nature of your spirit. You did not come here to live their life; you are here to live your own. The only expression you can live is your own. Good parents want one thing for their children—to be happy.

As you do The Practice, one day down the line, you will run into your parents' influence of energy within you, and when it dissolves, you will not find a sadness as their influence leaves but an openness to the happiness they wished all along for you.

Physical touch is only as beautiful
as your ability
to feel it from your heart.

Your brain feels through
physical touch

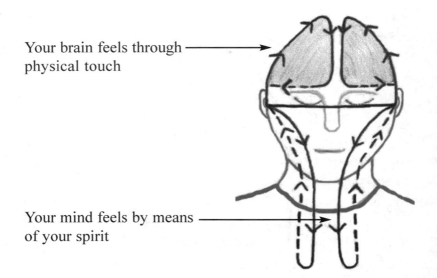

Your mind feels by means
of your spirit

There are two forms of feeling: one associated with the physical body and the other associated with the mind i.e., spirit.

If someone touches you and it feels cold and sterile, you have been touched by someone who is operating from his or her head. This cold feeling is a need to get and comes from destitution. This person is not in touch with the true nature of their being.

If someone touches you and you feel warmth, you have been touched by another's spirit. This warm feeling is the feeling of openness and love, a person who is living from their heart and not their head.

If you pay attention with your feeling sense when you are around people, you will notice you have two forms of feeling—physical and spiritual touch. Pay close attention to the deeper feeling sense from your heart in your greater Kelee, this is a beginning lesson in trusting your perception. The feeling sense of your spirit is something that starts out as a basic gut level feeling but leads into a deeper awareness that starts the process of opening the spiritual eyes of your soul.

It is important to know both ends of the human spectrum, harmony and disharmony. Watch carefully when you get a bad feeling about something, it is a warning! Also, watch carefully when you get a good feeling, there is something wonderful to experience.

When what we think and feel
are different,
it's called a mixed message.

When your brain thinks
one way

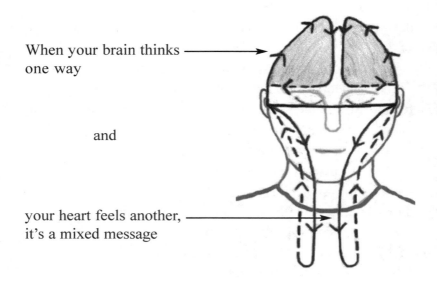

and

your heart feels another,
it's a mixed message

There are two mixed messages you need to be aware of: yours and another's.

Mixed messages begin when your head does not want to look at what your heart feels. If you don't want to look at emotional pain inside yourself, it's because you fear it or are ashamed of it—that's the reason you cover it up. This pain is a block to you opening up to your spirit.

The most difficult mixed messages are associated with love. When someone hurts another and says, "I love you," it is not love. Love never hurts. If you believe that this is love, you will love that which will hurt you, and fear that which will help you. When your conception of love compartmentalizes this way, you will unconsciously attract hurtful situation after hurtful situation to you. If you don't deal with your mixed message compartments, you may install them in another, and the confusion is passed on to someone else.

When someone gives you a mixed message, their words and the vibration surrounding what they say do not match. This is always when *something does not feel right.* Trust what you sense! A mixed message compartment perceives life backward, and so it feels backward. There is an old adage about evil: it's only live spelled backwards. Evil is a misperception of life and simply a mistake made on one's pathway to enlightenment.

As you get still through The Practice, clarity will show you what's what. Remember, everything is workable with The Practice, persistence and patience.

Your spirit opens you up,
compartments close you down.

The compartments of ——→
closers shut people down

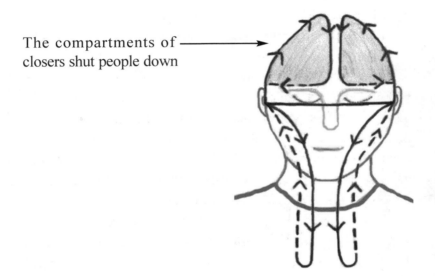

In life, there are people who invite you to open up and people who close you down.

If you're associating with people who operate from a need to always be right, they will close you down mentally. These individuals need you to feel less than them so they can appear more than you. This is of course ego. This small mind activity is governed by the animalistic behavior of survival of the fittest, which means someone has to be top dog. If two people want to be top dog, a confrontation happens, or worse, a fight. People who are closers don't want to look at their issues because on some level they fear themselves to be inferior. Ironically, they're already inferior but don't know it because they are living through inferior pervasive compartments. All compartments are inferior because they're not actually real.

If you have to protect yourself from a closer, you will have to protect yourself from them mentally. This forces your conscious awareness to be on guard, which should be a warning. Keep your distance from them. It is also extremely difficult to grow if you have to be in self-preservation mode. You cannot protect yourself and be open to deeper states of mind at the same time. The energy it will take to protect yourself from a closer will distract you from your own life experience. There is no faster way to be unlikeable than to be a closer. Even if a closer pretends to be nice, it's just as irritating; it's being fake. Pretending to live is not a form of living at all; it's a lack of courage to face fear.

When it comes to openers in life—no problem—openers are welcome anywhere.

The path you walk in life
is only dark
because you cannot see it clearly.

What you don't understand
about your mind can hurt you

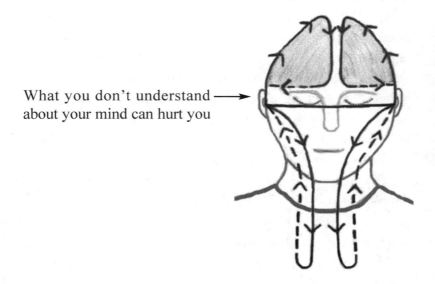

The Two Forms of Darkness

Darkness can appear in two basic ways: when you do not want to know what you see, and when you do not know what you see.

The first form of darkness is when you knowingly do not want to see. If you're knowingly deluding yourself and do not want to know you're doing it, who can help you? If you do not want to look at your own negative behavior, it's because you cannot face your own darkness from compartments within. If you find yourself in denial, it's because you cannot feel the beautiful openness of your spirit. If you knowingly had the choice to feel good or feel crappy, would you chose to feel crappy? It's the opposite of happy.

The second form is when you don't know what you see, this is the darkness of unknowing. This form of darkness is no more negative than nighttime is negative. The overall condition of the Kelee is just dark, unexplored, not negative.

Understanding your life can be a wonderful adventure, filled with new experiences that make you feel alive, if your mind is open to it. If you do walk into a situation because you're not paying attention and you pick up a painful compartment, this is the darkness of unknowing which will manifest as a mistake. Whether something has a harmonious or disharmonious outcome depends on your awareness level. This is the ongoing spiritual path.

Remember, *you give to yourself what you experience from life.*

*Personality
is a pattern of who you would like to be.
Self-expression
is an unobstructed experience
of who you really are.*

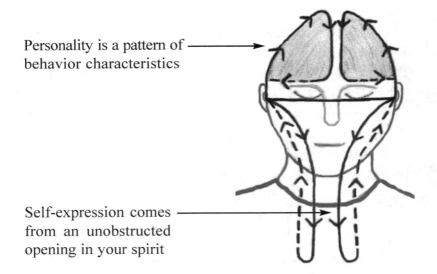

Personality is a pattern of
behavior characteristics

Self-expression comes
from an unobstructed
opening in your spirit

A definition of personality right out of the Random House Dictionary is: the visible aspect of one's character as it impresses others.

If you have ever noticed someone who has a strong personality, you will notice that they're always engaging you, whether you like it or not. For instance, when someone says, "Don't I look good?" This is because on some level they're looking for validation. If a pattern otherwise known as a compartment is controlling you, it is personality, not your spirits' self-expression.

Have you ever noticed that someone who has self-expression tends to be content without the need for recognition? This is always when they are secure within themselves naturally. For instance, let's say we consider a singer to be soulful. They have an unobstructed access to their spirit. They have no blocks i.e., compartments, to their self-expression. This is when you can feel their openness as it touches your soul. This form of self-expression is always unique, impressive and admired.

As you do The Practice and dissolve compartments, you will change out of a personality trying to be someone, into the self-expression of who you really are, from your spirit.

Become the person you are, and you will not need to be the person you should be.

*If you have to take
your independence,
you never really had it.*

Dependence comes from
attachments in the Kelee

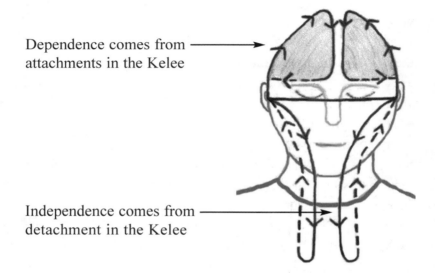

Independence comes from
detachment in the Kelee

Dependence and Independence

If someone is dependent on others, it is because they do not know how to operate from their mind i.e., spirit. To some degree all humans are dependent on each other for one thing or another. You probably don't make your clothes, grow your food, or didn't build your house. If you have the means to purchase these things—no problem—but if you steal or cheat to get things—big problem. If you cannot care for yourself by society's standards, you are not using your mind properly.

Whenever you attach to people or things, you form dependency. These attachments form compartments, which need energy to survive, which forms dependency. If you do not have the energy to feed your own compartments, you will pull energy mentally from others causing a dependency on others.

When it comes to independence in the material world, you may have material wealth, but that does not mean you will feel free with it. If you have attachments to money and things, you will worry about them. You can only escape your attachments when you are free from them by detaching from within your spirit.

If you are truly independent, you are not a burden on the outside world or to yourself. As you connect to your spirit through The Practice, you will become more independent and less dependent.

Remember, *fit into yourself and you will fit in anywhere.*

It's amazing,
when you don't do things to people,
they like it.

Unsolicited advice is another ⟶
name for a control issue i.e.,
compartment

There is no faster way to irritate someone than to offer unsolicited advice!

Advice works best when asked for!

Who wants to be told what to do with their life?

Good advice may have worked for you, but do you need to give it?

As you begin doing The Practice and your perception opens, you start seeing things other people do not see. Inevitably a dilemma arises. Do you say something about a problem that you see in another with your newly developed awareness? Do you offer advice when others do not want to see?

When you feel you must give your knowledge, watch that it isn't a control issue on your part. If you have some wisdom to impart, share how you solved a problem; don't tell others what to do. Perceived knowledge is for you! You are not required to share your knowledge. In addition, anytime you take credit for another's accomplishment because of your insight, you take away another's experience to feel good about learning. Take away someone's decision-making process and you have hindered, not helped. No one owns knowledge or wisdom!

Good advice is telling people how you would do something, not how they should do it. You help others most when you let them learn for themselves.

Remember, everyone ultimately must live life as they see fit through personal experience of mind.

Self-worth
is measured by how you live your life,
not by how others
think you should live.

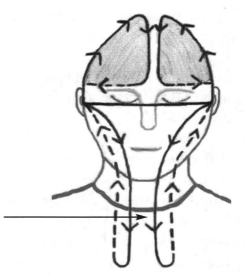

Self-worth comes from
your spirit not your head

You do not need another's opinion to have your own opinion of you. You are the only one who can decide how to live your life. If you listen to how others say you should live your life, you don't live your life, you live theirs. This is an inevitable regret ending with resentment. If you are living from a loving space, what's for another to say? If you're living from a negative space, that's for you to change, not someone else.

In the world there are philosophies that actually teach that you are not worthy from birth. This is a spiritual crime to teach someone they are not worthy. Do not believe it! It is impossible to feel good about yourself if at your deepest point in your conscious awareness you feel unworthy because of a misperception of you.

Who can decide your self-worth other than you? Who can feel worthy for you?

Everyone's spirit is beautiful by nature; you just have to get to it buried under negative compartments. How you find the real you ultimately comes from a feeling, a sense of worthiness within your heart found within your Kelee.

Each time you do The Practice, you dissolve what isn't you and get back to what is. It is actually quite easy to know who is the real you. It's the beautiful feeling in yourself.

Your spirit is worthy of any dream you can possibly dream.

The safe zone
with spiritual growth
is when you are open to it.

When you hide from your
issues, you never feel safe
from them

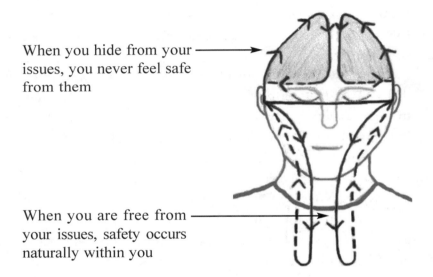

When you are free from
your issues, safety occurs
naturally within you

In life, there can be real danger and then there is the illusion of it.

When it comes to feeling safe in your life, you can feel safe physically but not within your mind, if you still fear life. This ability to feel safe within the mind is a real dilemma for many people because they do not really know how to face their fear and release it. It is no wonder why we fear, many of the issues i.e., comparments, that end up in the Kelee are stronger than your conscious awareness. This can be a real intimidation!

If you are avoiding your fears within i.e., compartments, can you really feel safe?

When you start doing The Practice, one of the first things you will face is what you have been avoiding all along. This will take practice, persistence and patience. You will hear this phrase many times and it is for good reason, to not forget what will see you through the difficult times of processing out compartments. When you do The Practice, you shift the balance of power from the brain to the mind. This happens naturally over time as the compartmentalized fear will be replaced by the space of your spirit in your Kelee.

When you truly understand the mind and know the right steps to take on your spiritual path of realization, *the truth will set you free.*

*When you are inspired to find,
you most assuredly will.*

Motivation is a generation
of energy from the head

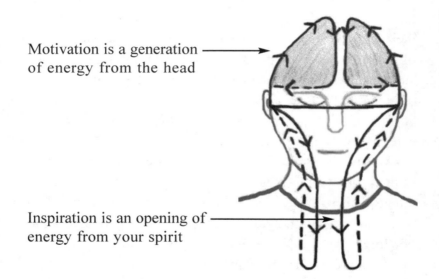

Inspiration is an opening of
energy from your spirit

When it comes to motivation and inspiration, they are two different forms of energy.

Motivation is electrochemical energy you must generate from the brain and it is always short lived. This electrochemical energy is available to your conscious awareness to do something but not necessarily with any great forethought. You are ready and willing to go but not sure where. You have good intentions but no wisdom. There is a famous phrase about this, "The road to hell is paved with good intentions." Motivation is energy to do, but lacks inspiration from your being i.e., spirit. Motivation works at its finest when it is directed by the spirit.

When it comes to inspiration, you don't have to generate energy to produce an effect in the world. You will notice, when you are truly inspired, it seems to come out of nowhere. This place is the space of your spirit, it's non-physical and a universal energy source.

Actually there are two forms of inspiration: from your own mind i.e., spirit, or from another's mind i.e., spirit, imparted to you. If you can't find inspiration in a time of need—ask. We all have loved ones watching out for us in the spiritual realm, whether we are aware of it or not. You may end up being inspired in a unique and beautiful way.

Your spirit
cannot be damaged,
even with everything you do to it.

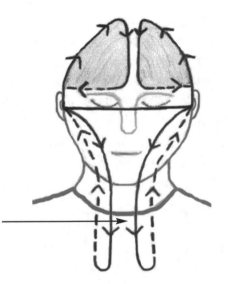

The best help you can give
yourself is when you are
quiet here

The saving grace for humanity is that with everything you do to hurt your spirit, it's all temporary. Your spirit is non-physical; you can do nothing to damage it permanently. You can cause yourself enormous amounts of emotional pain and abuse your physical body, but eventually you will learn from your mistakes one way or another.

To be harmonious, you must know how you hurt yourself versus how you help yourself. Ignorance promotes pain, awareness promotes growth.

Here are a few simple ways to help your life:

1. You help yourself the most by doing The Practice. Your mind i.e., spirit, is where all answers to all questions are realized! It's ironic that you wash the outside of your body daily but do not think to clean what's running it.

2. Drink pure water. In the morning fill up a half-gallon container of pure water and drink it by day's end. Water cleanses the body and is a necessary conductor of energy.

3. Most people do not need to eat as much as they do. Eat slower and less. Moderation is the key here. Food is fuel for the body, be mindful, eat healthy pesticide-free food and you'll feel better.

4. Exercise your body. Your body needs movement. Get into an exercise program. Explore your body's needs. This basic knowledge is out there already. Don't negate your body, enjoy it.

Most of what you need to heal yourself is to stop causing your own suffering. Your body is the vehicle for your spirit, take care of it and it will serve you well.

*How you learn
isn't from
what you already know,
it's from
what you don't know.*

Chapter Three

Your Conscious Awareness

*It is
the close observation
of your mind
that ultimately yields
its secrets.*

If you don't have your own perception
of life,
you won't have any.

Your conscious awareness
can operate in brain function

Your conscious awareness
can operate in dysfunction
from compartments

Your conscious awareness
can operate in mind function

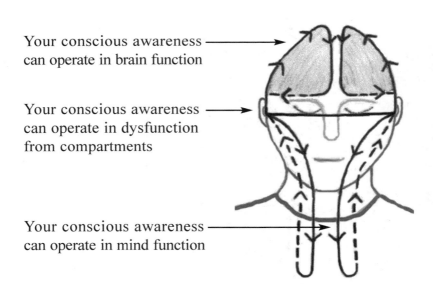

Your conscious awareness is a term that describes how consciously aware you are in each given moment. Your conscious awareness is what is reading this page right now; with each person's conscious awareness operating at different levels of awareness according to their life experience.

Without training, the conscious awareness operates in the intellect because society teaches us what to think but not necessarily how to think and certainly not how to feel. If we are to be consciously aware, knowledge must not be believed before our understanding of it.

What is more important, knowledge or wisdom? You may have knowledge and intelligence but not know what to do with it. Intelligence without wisdom is often a step before stupidity.

The conscious awareness without training tends to wander—commonly called daydreaming—and spreads out into occupational space. This means your conscious awareness is taking up space in your mind, but not necessarily functioning with any high degree of efficiency. If you want your conscious awareness to be perceptive, you must understand what's affecting it from within and what's distracting it from without.

It would be wise to understand what your conscious awareness is doing at all times. Remember, *you can only experience life in one place, and that's within your own mind.*

There is no greater perception
than your own clear one.

The beauty of pure perception →
is that it always presents life
correctly

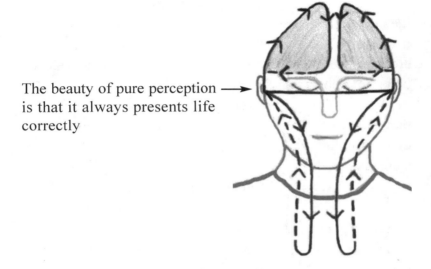

If you decide what you want to see before you see, you don't. As your mind stops being distracted by ego, chatter from the brain and compartments in your Kelee, your perception begins to develop.

The main reason perception is blocked is invariably due to compartments. When you can't accept the truth of what you see, you block what you see or change what you see to make yourself feel comfortable. The sad thing about compartments is you'll never see clearly if you don't know they're blocking your sight. The problems will relentlessly keep coming until you see what's really happening and make the right choices to end the suffering you're trying to escape. If you're trying to escape your own mind, where can you go, where your mind isn't?

Remember, *how truthfully you live is much better than believing you are truthful.* The truth is always simple when you see it, complex when you don't. The truth is always a clear perception of what is, not what you want the truth to be.

What everyone really wants to find in life doesn't need to take a lot of effort, if you have clear perception. If you are to develop your perception, you must start using it. This happens naturally as your conscious awareness starts using the observing space of mind function.

As a wise teacher once said to me, "If you see a beautiful lake and enjoy its presence, do you need someone to tell you, you are?"

*If you look to another
for your life,
you will only find someone else.*

Another's perception of you ⟶
is not yours of yourself

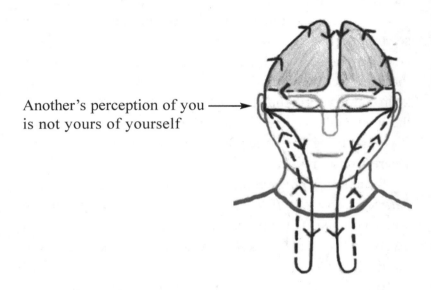

In life, it is certainly easier to follow another because it appears to be safer. What if you believe someone else's perception and they're wrong? How do you know anything except what you see from your own mind?

The true meaning of life isn't given by others. If you believe without the ability to see for yourself, you're blind; hence the term "blind faith." If you're worried about how others judge you, it's their judgment not yours. If you are learning and growing to the best of your ability, who is to judge?

At the most fundamental level, this is where The Practice starts clearing your conscious awareness to see for yourself the true condition of your life. When your conscious awareness learns to detach and is in a clear space in your mind, you see clearly. Amazingly enough, when each person sees clearly, we all see the same thing. As a wise man I know once said, "An elephant is an elephant, no matter what you call him."

One day, we will all agree that if you hurt another human being, it is wrong. If we cannot see this simple truth with our own individual perception, suffering will eventually drive anyone who does not yield to this most basic lesson.

You have the right to live life as you see fit, even if others don't like it, as long as you do not interfere with others. Is this not enough leeway in life to live peacefully?

The surface of the mind
is your reception point
to the world.

The electrochemical surface ——→
of the mind

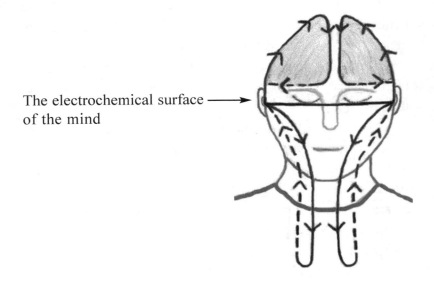

If you feel where your thoughts are right now, you will feel your thoughts at eye level. This is the electrochemical surface of the mind and with a little practice you will become familiar with it.

The surface of the mind is a reception point to the outside world; it is where your conscious awareness is right now reading this. It is an electrochemical plane of energy that splits between the pupils of your eyes, moves around the outside of your brain and down in between both hemispheres of your brain. The surface of the mind is a delineation between the outside physical world of sense-consciousness and the inside world of your spirit.

There are many common phrases that people use without really thinking about what they mean such as: *I have something weighing on my mind*—a compartment that is burdening you on the surface of your mind. *I have something on the back of my mind*—a compartment that's sitting on the back of the surface of your mind. *I can't get something off my mind*—a bothersome compartment that's distracting you and won't go away. All of these phrases will have a deeper, more real meaning when you begin doing The Practice. You will begin to understand your mind from the inside out. This will forever change your life in a beautiful fulfilling way.

The Practice will teach you once and for all how to free yourself from the weight on your mind that everyone would so like to drop.

Awakening
is not always controlled by what you see,
but many times
by what you don't.

Compartments can be installed, ⟶
self-created, or pervasive

Awakening

When you start The Practice, you will start the process of awakening. How can you enlighten your mind if you're unaware of how to do it?

As your mind calms down and you wake up, you'll notice your mind has formed compartments in three basic ways: compartments installed from others, self-created compartments and pervasive compartments from society.

Installed compartments are installed by people around us and are triggered by them or people who remind us of them. These compartments force you to acknowledge your behavior, so you must deal with them first. Ironically, it's your family or close friends who press most of your buttons because they installed them. Those who are closest to you can get to you the easiest.

Self-created compartments are the next layer of compartments you'll become aware of. These compartments you create to make you feel good about yourself. They can be comfort zones, belief systems or fear of potential fear. These compartments you must root out yourself.

Pervasive compartments are the hardest to find because they are ingrained in you as cultural behavior—how to be from others, the media, advertising and every other influence that makes you other than yourself. Because you live through these compartments, becoming aware of them takes a great deal of detachment. If you really want to be free, you must be free from all conditioning to see things the way they really are, not how the world would have you see.

When it comes to understanding life, *if you really see, you'll get it, if you don't, you won't*.

If you see
what you want to see,
you don't see
what you're looking at.

You don't see outside yourself, →
without first seeing from inside
yourself

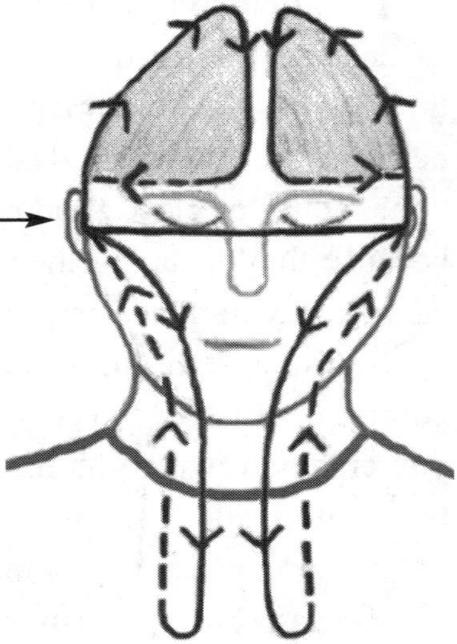

If you want to understand life, you must learn to see it as it really is. Why do we not see life as it really is?

Ego wants to see only what it wants to see. If you are insecure with yourself, you create an ego. The ego is a self-creation of you, not the true nature of who you really are. Ego decides before it perceives, so it cannot see other than what it has predetermined as reality. Ego is only a temporary replacement for what you don't understand about yourself. Ego is a substitute for mind function. If you feel good about yourself, do you need an ego?

Compartments filter incoming information from the outside world. Compartments are another of the big blocks to seeing clearly in the world. All compartments are fear-based and all fear is a block in the mind. If you don't want to look at something in your own mind, you will not want to look at the equivalent in the outside world. As you do The Practice and the compartments dissolve in your mind, the space occupied by the compartment will be replaced with your spirit. When you see with clarity from your spirit, life is perceived in a real way.

Missing spiritual puzzle pieces represent the absence of experience. You cannot be faulted for not knowing what you have not experienced; this is the reason for living. You do not need to feel bad about what you don't know about yourself. When you open to your spirit and find missing puzzle pieces, what was once a problem or misperception is now understanding from clear perception. The need to change reality to fit your insecure comfort zones is not necessary anymore. You become at ease with reality and allow it to be only what it is.

When we do not try
to experience life
is when we always do.

The brain operates through
hard effort

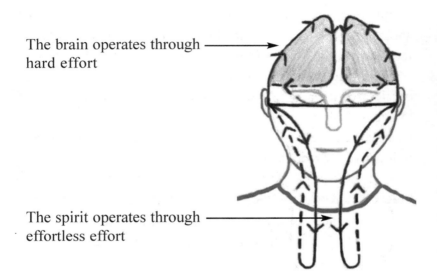

The spirit operates through
effortless effort

When it comes to how your conscious awareness operates there's hard trying and there's effortless effort. Trying is energy going outward. Experience is energy coming inward.

How many times have you racked your brain, looking for an answer? This is always when you were trying too hard to troubleshoot a problem. When you finally give up in frustration and are ready to quit, the answer mysteriously pops into your head. If the answer didn't come from your brain, it came from your mind i.e., spirit.

When you try too hard, you get in your own way. Have you ever heard the phrase, "Don't try so hard"? We know this to be true, but how do you try to not try? Use less energy in your brain and more energy will shift into your mind i.e., spirit. It's not necessary to drive your brain at one hundred miles an hour, slow down and your spirit will enjoy the ride.

The brain uses a hard form of analytical energy and the mind i.e., spirit, uses a soft, subtle form of energy. The hard form of electrochemical energy is for running our body's organic system, and the soft subtle form of energy is for running our spirit. It is these two forms of energy that bond the physical and spiritual together. When the electrochemical bond is broken, the physical experience ends and the spirit is released into the spirit realm.

Remember, the intricacies of our spirit flow when we do not try to force our life experience.

*Conserving energy
is a wise man's
understanding of it.*

Energy itself does not bring
success, awareness does

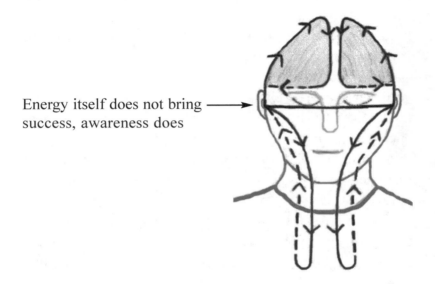

There are many situations in life that after close observation, you will realize are better to stay out of. Anytime you expend energy, you will also expend time. If you're operating by random firing neurons from the brain, you will waste energy because of a lack of awareness from your mind i.e., spirit. You only have a limited supply of energy from your brain; it would be wise to know what you do, before you do it.

As you begin to calm yourself, you will start to understand a new range of energy within your mind. This range of energy extends from the electrochemical energy of the brain to the universal form of energy in your spirit. When your conscious awareness operates from your spirit, you expend less energy and perceive with more clarity and less fragmentation. As you begin to do The Practice, you'll become aware of how much time and energy you waste because of fruitless actions.

Have you ever noticed, if you're in a hurry, you're coming from your brain? If you're patient, you're coming from your mind i.e., spirit. When your spirit is directing your brain, you will not waste energy needlessly. Your mind i.e., spirit, operates through an observation mode, which can save you a lot of time and energy.

When you're living in the universal energy of your spirit, free from the constraints of the outside world, it feels as if an angelic benefactor is paying you to live your life; it's an amazing feeling of freedom. I highly recommend it.

The light of awareness
illumines
the depths of your soul.

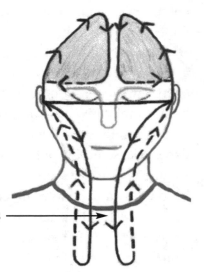

The light of awareness appears
as clarity in your Kelee

The Light of Awareness

When you start doing The Practice and begin to still your conscious awareness, the light of your awareness begins to brighten. This happens naturally as your conscious awareness moves into the feeling sense of mind function, which is the observing part of you. As this happens, you begin to detach from the chattering brain function and the dysfunction from compartments distracting you.

As you continue to do The Practice, your conscious awareness becomes more sensitive as it calms down. Your sensitivity will ultimately become your perception. This will begin the process of opening the spiritual eyes of your soul or your mind's eye. Whatever darkness you had previously taken in, the light of awareness will now illuminate. As your light of awareness grows brighter, you grow mentally stronger.

When you shine a light into a dark place, you cease to fear the darkness. Then you can begin to understand the grand illusion of compartments; they are misperceptions of life that were leading you astray. The ability to see clearly brings confidence; this turns into self-assurance and deeper states of knowing. When your conscious awareness brightens, so will the inside of your Kelee. It is from the light of your awareness that you see where you are going on your path. Remember, your spiritual path is about you; it's your personal relationship with life.

We are all beings unto our own light. Brighten yourself and the world brightens around you.

Awareness
is openness to life
without fear.

Awareness is an understanding
of what your conscious
awareness perceives

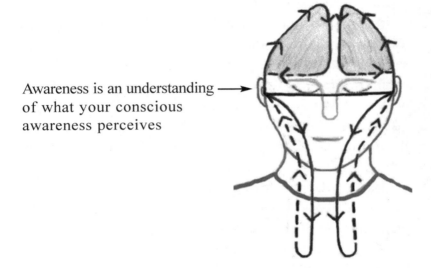

The brain remembers but it takes the mind to understand. In other words, the brain only knows what the mind has understood first, from experience.

How many times have you read something, remembered what you read, but still can't make sense of it? You have the data but not the understanding. If you believe the written word before you understand it, do you understand or just think you understand? If you say, "I think I know." You don't. You're still thinking about it.

The brain believes because it doesn't know. When the mind truly knows, it's not a belief. Awareness is the means by which you understand beyond belief.

If you're stubborn with your beliefs, you may defend them to your death because they represent you or what you think is you. Nothing truthful ever needs to be defended. It is what it is and will manifest what it is, good or bad. Truth is an understanding of harmony and disharmony. To see the truth, however, you must understand what blocks your awareness from the truth. The number one reason people do not see the truth is because of compartments i.e., fear-based blocks. If you see what you want to see, you don't see the truth. Get the blocks out of the way and your mind i.e., spirit, will see.

What keeps your awareness open? A still conscious awareness free from preconceived thoughts or beliefs.

*When your mind is bright
with the light of awareness,
no shadows can approach at all.*

Shadows are the negative
prelude of compartments

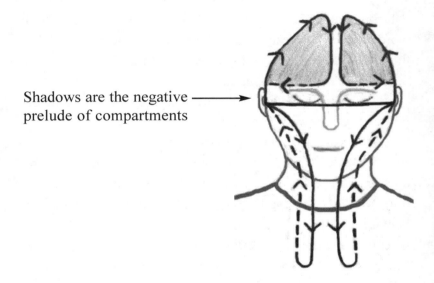

Nothing in life grows well in a shadow, so it would be wise to understand what they are. Shadows can come from two places: another's mind or your own.

When you meet someone for the first time and get a bad feeling, it's a warning. What you sense is from a compartment with an agenda. You are about to be compromised. It would be wise to move out of this shadow and in another direction as quickly as possible. This shadow is the precursor to compartmentalized fear. When you learn to see the shadows of compartments, you can keep yourself out of a lot of trouble. Remember, nobody's spirit is evil. The only evil in life comes from compartments; they're misperceptions of life and do things wrongly.

The other place a shadow can appear is within your own mind. Shadows can be intimidating and frightening. Nevertheless, how can you get away from what is within you? You can try to block them, but this makes you comfortable with being uncomfortable. Remember, a shadow coming from another can represent danger, but the shadows in your own mind are only the illusion of danger.

When you do The Practice and bring your mind to a still point in your greater Kelee, this point opens your mind to clear perception and becomes the light of awareness. The light of awareness will dispel the darkness of any shadow. When you can see the fear within for what it really is—misperception—you will stop fearing shadows once and for all.

Being brave
isn't blocking out fear,
it's being able to look at it.

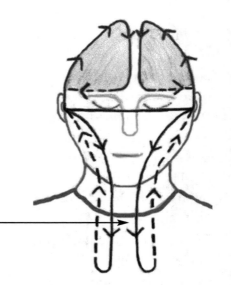

You cannot escape from
where you must come
home to, your spirit

The hardest thing you will ever do in your life will be to face your fear within. If your fear i.e., compartments, is stronger than you are, what do you do?

Compartmentalized fear is always the reason people escape reality. Escaping problems only results in an empty feeling of mere existence.

As you begin to do The Practice, your conscious awareness will strengthen as your compartments weaken, with the balance of power shifting in your favor. It's a wonderful thing to feel free from compartments. As you have more free time, your awareness begins to open to other areas of your mind. The strength you have been building is in preparation for an inevitable happening, you come up against something big! An issue you do not want to look at is facing you. What do you do? You have been trained through The Practice to not avoid your compartments, but the fear is stronger than your conscious awareness. If there is a test in life, this is it! You may try to go back to how you used to be, but you can't, you're not that person anymore. You're between a rock and a hard place. As a master said to me many years ago, "There are still some dark areas in your mind, explore them bravely. When your mind has the light of awareness, no shadows can approach at all."

When you learn to open to your spirit, you will never be without courage again!

*It's not
what you convince yourself of
that's real,
it's what really is!*

The root of delusion is
conscious awareness
misperception

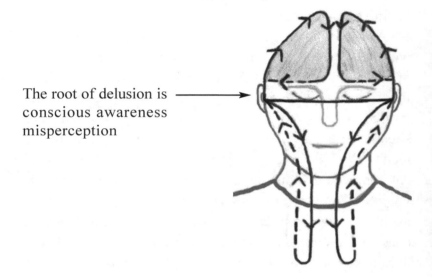

Delusion is not an easy subject to face and yet if you don't, you're always facing the wrong direction in life.

Delusion can happen in three basic ways:

1. **You see what you want to see.** When you cannot tell the difference in your mind, between the way things are and your own self-creation, there's trouble. Trouble is always the fragmentation of the truth. When delusion from self-created ego is stronger than reality, the delusion appears real. If what you don't want to see outside you is reminding you of your own inferiority, you will see what you want to see regardless of the consequences, and most often at the expense of others.

2. **Your conscious awareness is colored by the negativity of compartments.** In this case, you're not intentionally deluding yourself; compartments are coloring what you're seeing and you're not aware of it. You may have good intentions, but still are not seeing things the way they actually are, hence the phrase, "The road to hell is paved with good intentions."

3. **Your spirit does not have the knowledge to know what you're looking at.** This is when at the deepest level of your spirit, you do not have the knowledge to see what you're looking at because you haven't had the experience to know differently. You have missing spiritual puzzle pieces. You may make mistakes, but you will learn eventually, as you find those elusive spiritual puzzle pieces, that one day will end all delusion once and for all.

If you're not in your mind,
you're out of it.

The mind i.e., spirit, occupies
the space of the lesser and
greater Kelee

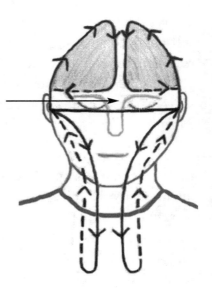

Mind Function

To understand the mind, we must understand it through practicality, not theory. Within all of us are two distinct parts, brain function and mind function. Brain function is associated with the thinking process, memory and the intellect. Mind function is associated with perception, the feeling process, awareness and the spirit. The two can work as one but there tend to be conflicts between what we think and feel. This ends up being the big mind/small mind battle for domination.

When we hear the word "mindful," it denotes a mind that is aware and comprehends. When we hear the expression, "You're out of your mind," it's when the wisdom of mind function i.e., spirit, is not present. As you begin to do The Practice, you will become increasingly familiar with mind function. You begin to realize that the brain through sense consciousness only brings information to you, but it takes the mind to understand it.

Mind function actually operates through both spaces of the lesser and greater Kelee. The lesser and greater Kelee are actually the same space. However, it's only from extended practice that you can operate from the space in the lesser Kelee area without being overruled by the brain, because most people's heads rule their hearts.

Over time, from The Practice you will move your conscious awareness increasingly from the small mind i.e., brain, into the big mind i.e., spirit. It is an evolution of understanding called a spiritual path and that of finding enlightenment, the crown jewel of humanity.

Nothing exists without your mind's awareness of it.

*Analyzation
is a process of the brain,
while observation
is a process of the spirit.*

Analyzation is the intellectual
process of the brain

Observation is the understanding
process of the spirit

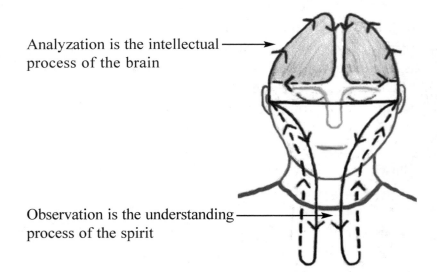

Analyzation and Observation

The analyzation process of the brain is marvelous when it works properly. Problems occur when the conscious awareness runs into blocks called compartments; it gets frustrated when it searches for what it can't find.

The brain is extremely complex and needs simplification to run smoothly. The brain is good at examining the linear world, but when it comes to the emotions, it flounders because they seem to be illogical. Try finding resolution to a relationship issue with the intellect and you'll find real frustration. The brain deals well with things, but not with people.

The most beautiful way to live is through the observation process of the spirit. The spirit can bypass the intellect's analyzation process and see without predetermining how you should live. The spirit can have an unobstructed view of life if it doesn't have compartments in the way.

Unfortunately, the analyzation and observation process are both subject to the problems associated with compartments. However, as you do The Practice, you set into motion the undoing of what is not helping you—your compartments.

When analyzation and observation work together, it's amazing! Pay attention to both processes and you will learn something about two different worlds, the one within and the one without.

*Finding yourself
does not require anything
other than your own reception of you.*

Clear reception is an
unobstructed conscious
awareness

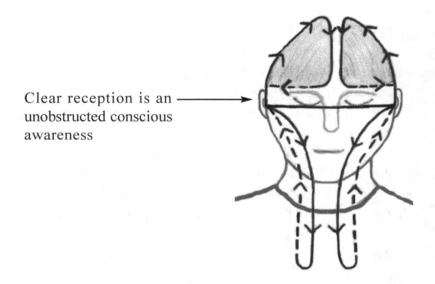

Receptivity

If you're living from your outward senses i.e., brain/ intellect, you will be forever looking outside yourself in something other than your spirit to find yourself. The brain only knows how to look at the outside world, but not into your spiritual world. The brain is good with seeing matter but not with seeing the energy of thought and how the mind really works.

Do you know why your mind is not receptive sometimes?

To unravel why your reception to life is blocked, you must understand compartmentalized fear. To start, this will take being comfortable with your conscious awareness. But to troubleshoot your mind, you will need to attain a detached unobstructed conscious awareness.

Whether we are talking about reception of incoming information from the outside world or reception of incoming information from your inside world, stillness is important for clarity.

When your mind slows down, reception accelerates; this is extremely important in understanding the deeper points of your mind i.e., spirit. Each time you still your mind in The Practice your reception becomes less obstructed, but it will take patience to master, as with anything of value.

Remember, *when everything goes out, nothing comes in.* Receptivity is about allowing what you see to come in unaltered from wherever, not determining what you see before you do.

Allow yourself to be receptive and you will be amazed at what there is to receive.

Our spiritual reflection
comes not from our physical nature,
but how we see
from our spiritual nature.

Our eyes reflect back our
physical presence

Our spirit reflects back our
spiritual presence

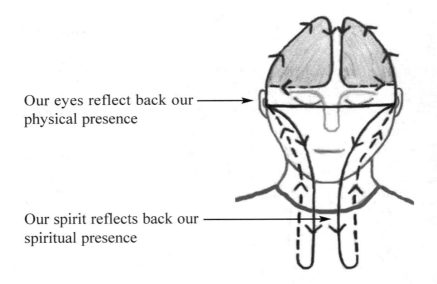

The metaphor of a reflecting pond has long been used to help people sit still and look within to understand their thoughts, but how to do this?

If you are to understand spiritual reflection, you must move beyond your physical eyes. Your physical eyes can see outside yourself, but it's your spiritual eyes that see inside yourself. Your physical eyes collect what you see, but your spiritual eyes makes sense of it. How you see your true reflection is not how you see physically, but how you see spiritually.

As you do The Practice and get out of brain function and into mind function, you begin to truly see. If you feel lost, it's always because you don't understand what you see. Whether you're looking outside yourself or inside yourself, you must learn to know what you see. You must learn to trust in your perception, if you are to understand yourself.

Right now, your conscious awareness is at the surface of your mind; feel down inside your greater Kelee, what do you feel? This is how you start to see your reflection, you may feel emotional pain or you may feel love. Whatever you feel is the way to understand what is and what isn't you. Beautiful feelings are you, painful ones are not.

Study what's reflected back to your conscious awareness and you will learn many things about the art of self-reflection and why you are, the way you are.

The Kelee
is the proverbial
fountain of youth.

Your brain takes energy ⟶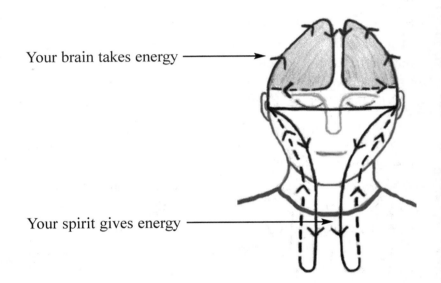

Your spirit gives energy ⟶

If you look at the Kelee diagram closely, you'll notice that it's the energy from your spirit that gives to your head. *Your spirit gives energy, while your head takes energy.*

If you experience your life without feeling your spirit, your life will feel empty because it has no depth. If you can't open to the energy of your spirit, you'll need to overcompensate by getting energy from somewhere. If you want fulfillment in your life, you must open to your spirit. It's how you become young at heart and open to the wonder the world has to offer.

Explore that which touches you, and you will find that which does.

Remember, it's the heart of your spirit that brings meaning to your head; your brain only files the memories from experiences. The Kelee diagram shows how your spirit feeds your brain with energy. Without the spirit, the body will not run. Without a physical body, life in the physical as we know it does not exist. The lesser and greater Kelee together make up the Kelee, the union of body and mind i.e., spirit.

If you look at the diagram closely, you'll notice that the Kelee is actually an inverted fountain of energy folding in upon itself. Do The Practice and you will open to the proverbial fountain of youth. It is real and within you already, you just need to find it.

The fountain of youth
is found
in how you feel,
not how you look.

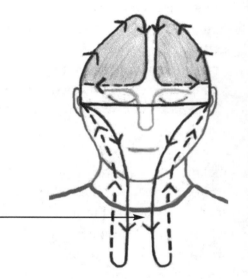

The fountain of youth is
found in your spirit

It has long been known that people who are happier, live longer and healthier lives. The question would then be, if you're not happy, why aren't you?

The number one reason for unhappiness and aging prematurely is stress and worry from compartments. Compartments are negative-based energy patterns that draw energy from your electrochemical energy. Compartments pull energy from your physical body thus aging you through a form of malnutrition of your soul. Have you ever noticed that when someone has a worried look on their face, they look older?

As humans, we are a physical and spiritual creature together. The Practice will slow the aging process to a rate that will be in harmony with your DNA structure. If you want to age slower, live from the wisdom of your spirit not the recklessness of your brain. When you're living mostly from your brain, you will always be concerned with time because your brain lives in a linear state. If you want to experience more time, slow your pace so you can live more in your mind i.e., spirit. If you're moving too fast, you age fast, so what's the point? Let's speed up life and die quicker?

If you're concerned about how you look, take a look at how you feel. A warm, loving heart will do wonders in the aging process. When you learn to live from your spirit, you will live where there is no old. Your spirit does not have a body to age; it can feel young at any age.

Being *young at heart* is found by being in your Kelee where your spirit resides. If you want to find the fountain of youth, live in your own heart i.e., spirit.

*Boredom
is what steals life from you,
vibrancy
is what gives it back.*

Boredom is the brain's
absence of mindfulness

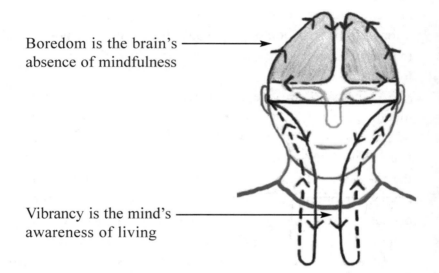

Vibrancy is the mind's
awareness of living

When you begin to do The Practice, your life will not become boring. You will not be so calm and mellow you won't want to do anything. This is what you will not experience through The Practice!

Being physical and having excitement is great, but it's only half of the human equation. What about the experience of contentment after excitement? You cannot always run around excited, you have to come down some time, either by running out of things to do, or by your energy crashing. If you run out of excitement and find yourself bored, you're living more from your brain, than your mind i.e., spirit.

The replacement for boredom is vibrancy; it's when the mind experiences the newness of life. This newness is the eternal moment of life everyone is looking to find.

If you look at the Kelee diagram and the surface of the mind, you will notice this is where the outside world meets your conscious awareness. If you take what comes to you and move it directly into memory, you have bypassed the feeling process and the vibrancy of life; this is what is considered the shallow experience of life. When you allow life experience to be felt through the greater Kelee and then filed into memory, you experience what is considered depth.

Shallow and bored is the lesser of us, deep and vibrant is the greater. It's your choice what you experience in your life, always!

*Fulfillment
is the acceptance
of what each moment
has to give.*

Temporary satisfaction comes
from the brain

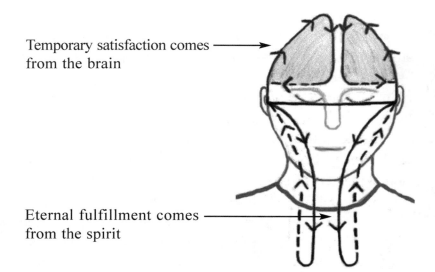

Eternal fulfillment comes
from the spirit

There are two basic ways to receive: from the outside world in what you do and from your inside world in who you are.

Accomplishments in life are great. But whenever you operate predominately from your head, the greatness tends to be short-lived, because as each moment moves on, your accomplishments are left behind. Your brain operates in a production-based way; it has to keep on the move to feel secure and in control. Your brain never feels like it has enough because it can only feel temporary satisfaction, not eternal fulfillment from your spirit.

Nothing outside us, by what we do, can be realized until our spirit is open to it.

Everything we do outside us is realized from within us first. If you don't know what to do, what ends up being done? If your mind i.e., spirit, does not precede what you do, you don't realize what you do. In fact, your spirit does not have to actually do something to feel good; your spirit can merely observe the world and enjoy being in it.

Some people believe if you're not driven, it means you're lazy, but it's quite the opposite. When you enjoy life, everything you do is naturally of a high quality, which comes back to you as a form of accomplishment.

Real fulfillment comes when you're aware of what you do by being open to your spirit in your Kelee.

*The only constraints
you have
are the ones
you have placed
upon yourself.*

Chapter Four

Compartments

*It's the simplicity
of stillness
that unravels the complexity
of compartments.*

*Compartments
are the garbage
of your soul.*

Compartments can
superimpose over the
brain

Compartments can
form on the surface
of the mind

Compartments can
be in the lesser and
greater Kelee

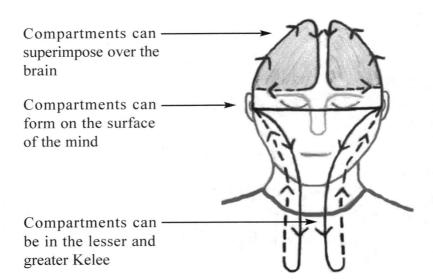

Compartments are called many names in our society: baggage, issues, buttons, dysfunction, and bullcrap, to name a few. When you're born up until this moment in time, energy from life experience is pouring through your mind. When you, not knowing any better, take in a negative thought-form image, it can become trapped in your Kelee as a compartment.

Compartments form when you take into your mind something that is not good for you, and you cannot let go of it. Compartments can form with or without you consciously knowing it. Negativity is everywhere in the world and can be directed at you with words or simply taken in as a bad feeling. In an event to stop yourself from feeling negative feelings once they have gotten inside you, you compartmentalize them to control them. Next, you have to start protecting yourself from the compartments with fear-based walls. Inadvertently you start feeding the compartments and make closed loop dysfunction.

Psychological malfunctioning is the garbage of humanity and has produced a disease on the planet called dysfunction—Compartmentism—a person who has little or no free space to operate in their mind. Compartments are misperceptions of who we are and separate us from our true nature and from the world we live in. The cure to rid this disease is here—it's called The Practice.

*Dysfunction
never takes a day off,
it doesn't even take a holiday.*

Your spiritual pond is the
Kelee, this is where
you jump in

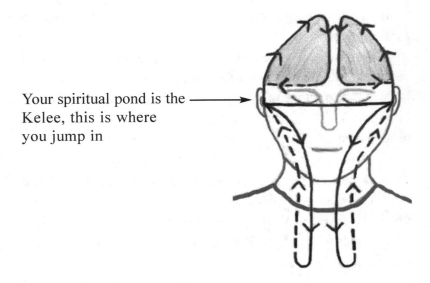

We operate in three basic ways: brain function associated with the body, mind function associated with the spirit, and dysfunction associated with misperception from compartments in the Kelee.

When dysfunction from compartments has been in your Kelee for a long time, it can leach into your conscious awareness and filter the beauty of life out. Think of your spirit as a beautiful pond and compartments as being garbage. When you learn through The Practice to clean out existing garbage and stop adding new garbage, your pond will clean up. Think of your conscious awareness as you in the pond. When the pond is clean, the pond will cleanse you. As your conscious awareness gets still in the greater Kelee, even the deepest dysfunction in your conscious awareness will eventually leach out of you.

There are many techniques trying to teach people how to swim. The Practice will teach you what you're swimming in and how to clean out the compartments. If your conscious awareness is to feel clean, compartments must be cleaned out of your spiritual pond i.e., Kelee. As your spiritual pond cleans up, so will you.

Each day can feel like a holiday when dysfunction is not in the way of a good time. When dysfunction is no longer at your expense, every day will be a good day. Give dysfunction the day off, do The Practice.

Compartments exist,
whether
you're aware of them or not.

Compartments are the ——————→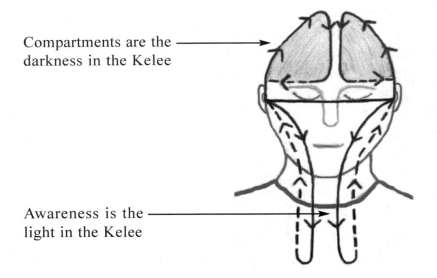
darkness in the Kelee

Awareness is the ——————
light in the Kelee

Compartments form in two basic ways: from outside circumstance or we create them.

When a compartment enters your mind from another, it's because you don't know how to stop it. You accept someone else's thought-form image into your mind; it doesn't feel like you, but it's in you and once in you, the confusion starts. If you cannot get into mind function and detach from the compartment, you may be unaware of the compartment's influence. Isn't it amazing that you could get mad and not even recognize you're angry? This is when a compartment has consumed you. This is a total lack of awareness.

The other form of compartments we create ourselves. If you create a compartment—which is a self-creation of life or a misperception of life—your conscious awareness will think the compartment is the real you, but in actuality it's not. It's easy to see how denial can happen. You would swear the behavior from the compartment is not you and in the true sense it's not, but the compartment still has a behavior of its own. It's amazing that everyone around may see what's going on but you. If your behavior acts on its own, who's doing it?

The Practice will open your spiritual eyes to compartmentalized behavior. How The Practice does this is through the light of awareness dispelling the darkness of unknowing. Awareness is the first step; detachment is the second step, with the third step being your freedom.

There is never
a valid reason
to abuse yourself.

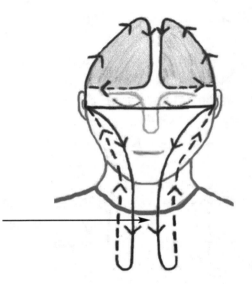

Self-abuse occurs when
you do not feel good
about who you are

To understand self-abuse issues, you must know how abuse originates.

1. **Self-abuse by sense-consciousness cravings.** When an abuse issue comes from a need to satisfy sense-consciousness cravings, it can become a physiological problem involving eating disorders, sexual issues and drug addictions, to name a few. The deeper problems stem from compartments and even deeper missing spiritual puzzle pieces. When you're in mind function, and not ruled by brain function or compartments, detachment occurs and sense-consciousness cravings are controlled.

2. **Self-abuse from a compartment.** If an abuse issue comes from a compartment, the compartment will have a negative perception of you. The abusive compartment formed because your mind believed a misperception that's now hurting you. When you dissolve the abusive compartment through The Practice, abusive behavior ends.

3. **Self-abuse by your conscious awareness turning on yourself.** Turning on yourself helps nothing. At the deepest level when your conscious awareness feels lost, it's because you're blocked from feeling by compartments, which leaves you disconnected from your spirit. You have issues because you have not learned the eternal lessons your spirit is seeking, namely finding your spiritual puzzle pieces.

When you don't understand your spirit, it leads to mental problems. When you don't understand your mental problems, it leads to physical problems. Every problem is related to your spirit, one way or another. The completion of your spirit is ultimately where all abuse ends.

Depression forms
when you turn
on yourself.

Depression can appear in —————
the lesser and greater Kelee

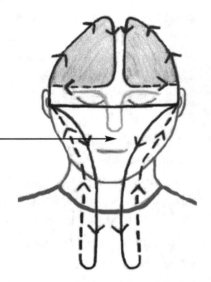

Depression is a hidden darkness in society and greatly misunderstood. Whenever you believe someone's negative opinion of you or you create one of your own, you form depression.

Depression appears in the Kelee as electrochemical thought-form images that have a thinking process independent of your conscious awareness. They always appear as dark spaces in forms such as: tar pits, black holes, quicksand or any dark nebulous space your mind can think of.

Depressive compartments are kept alive by you living through them or by your conscious awareness being angry with them. Turning on your compartments only makes them stronger.

When through The Practice you learn to detach from depression, you stop feeding it. Instead of you turning on the depression, the depressive compartment turns on itself, consuming itself until it has no more energy. When it's gone, you'll know it. You'll consciously search for it in your mind but it won't be there. As the distraction of the depressive compartment leaves, in its place is the open space of your spirit and the ability to clearly see why you see yourself so negatively. This is the point when realization can happen.

The deeper reason why depression forms is you still have missing spiritual puzzle pieces. You really can free yourself from forming depression by opening your spiritual eyes to that which will free you—self-realization—with the help of your mind i.e., spirit.

*Freedom is the ability
to exercise thought
without fear.*

Compartments in the Kelee ⟶
are another name for a jail cell

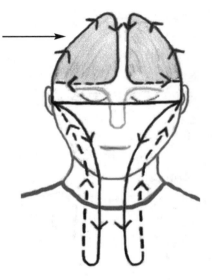

When you're afraid to experience life, it's because of fear in your mind. It's like going into a prison cell, closing the door and thinking you'll be safe but you're still in jail!

If you convince yourself you're safe in your compartments, you'll start becoming comfortable with being uncomfortable. This is how you start the process of being set in your ways. In actuality, you are set in compartments. If you start living through these compartments, you stop bringing in new information, which means you stop filing new memories. If you stop using your neuropathways of memory, they will shut down and finally you'll stop remembering. If you stop using your memory, what do you think happens? You have set into motion Alzheimer's! It's interesting to note that Alzheimer's usually starts after the age of sixty when a build-up of compartments happens. I have watched people of all ages actually re-open the pathways of memory by removing compartments.

If you're not able to move freely with your thoughts, you will be imprisoned by them. Remember, it's only the fear from unfortunate past events called compartments that block the doorway to experience. Compartments not only block your memory, but can also block the present and future moments to come.

Open the door of your mind with The Practice and you will walk out of the imprisonment of fearful compartments and into freedom of thought.

*Compartments are memories
that have not been accepted
as the past.*

Memories exist in
the brain network

Compartments exist in
the Kelee

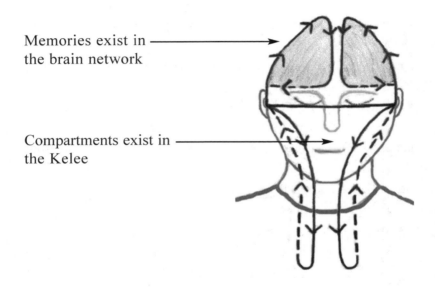

Memory and Compartments

When it comes to the past, it can be difficult to tell the difference between a memory and a compartment. A memory will exist only in the past, as the past. It is something that when you recognize it as such, you will know it cannot be changed. Memories are cast in stone! Kind of makes you want to be more careful with the moment, doesn't it?

A compartment exists as the past but still wants to change the present. Compartments are time capsules with an apparent mind of their own concerned with self-preservation. They will do just about anything to survive and they do so quite well unless you learn how to not feed them.

Compartments operate outside the view of sense-consciousness. They cannot be seen, unless you know how to see them with your spiritual eyes. People feel the effects of their negative behavior all the time but feel powerless to change them, so the compartments remain in the unseen world within the Kelee.

As you begin to do The Practice, you will begin to sense your compartments as you move through them in your practice. You will experience them as resistance or something that is hard to move through with your conscious awareness.

Understanding the difference between a memory and a compartment is just another level of awareness in the mind and the continuing way of freedom and enlightenment. Remember, memories exist in the brain, compartments in the Kelee.

*When you deny
your own dysfunction,
you protect
what you don't even like about yourself.*

Self-preservation compartments
are a confused form of survival ⟶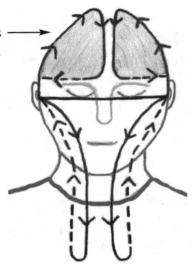

The hardest compartments to get rid of are self-preservation compartments. They're compartments that can defend themselves with justification and validation as to why they should exist.

Have you ever called someone on their compartment and they make you feel as if you're the one doing something wrong? They blame you for their dysfunction. If you can't deal with someone pointing out your dysfunction, it's quite common to blame another for pointing out your problem. Remember, blame is for the lame of mind. If you can't take responsibility for your dysfunction, you'll never get rid of it. A self-preservation compartment is hard on everyone but more importantly, on you; you're the one stuck with it.

It can be torturous having these compartments; they send thoughts of unworthiness to your conscious awareness, angering you with yourself for feeling them. You send anger back to the compartment, which feeds the compartment. Anger feeds anger, making closed loop dysfunction. A compartment that has no consciousness is keeping itself alive at your expense and you can't stop it. Who can get you out of this? Only you!

If you are to break these compartments, you must first be aware of the condition. Second, you must relax your conscious awareness so you can detach from the compartment; after all, the compartment is not really you. The Practice will take care of this dilemma by not feeding the compartment and breaking the compartment's self-preservation hold on you.

It takes no great skill to be angry;
however,
it takes great skill to control it.

Anger is an emotion of
protection or retaliation

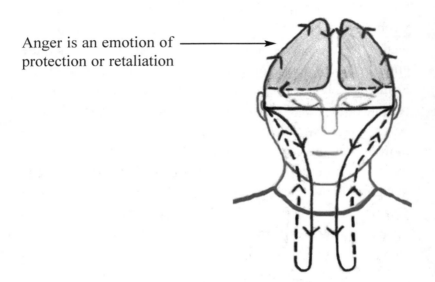

Anger is an emotion that can be used for protection or retaliation. Whenever we feel like we're being violated in some way, it is most likely that anger will be invoked. It is one thing to use anger for protection, but it's another if you use it to retaliate against another. If you retaliate, karma is set into motion with all of the cause and effect associated with disharmony. Are you sure you want to go down this path? If people can elicit anger in you, they can control you. There is an old saying, "He who angers you, controls you."

It is quite common in an effort to control angered frustration that your conscious awareness will compartmentalize your dissatisfaction. If the compartment of anger is stronger than your conscious awareness, you explode and probably install the same anger that's in you in another. You just passed your dysfunction to another and it may very well come back to haunt you.

Anger can compartmentalize in your conscious awareness, in the lesser Kelee, greater Kelee and on the surface of the mind. Anger can be a destructive energy; it's like having a live grenade in your hand with an explosion imminent, if you're not in control of your mind. When anger is no longer compartmentalized and you are in control of your mind, you will master the emotion of anger!

Once again, awareness is the ultimate form of protection. Awareness is the way to understand that retaliation is a double-edged sword, cutting you first with its disharmony.

When you're hot under the collar,
it's a compartment
producing the heat.

When compartments
are on fire, so are you

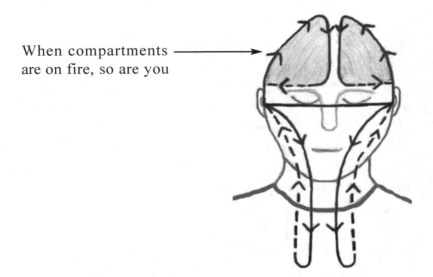

How many times have you heard someone say, "That burns me up," or "Man, am I steamed." These are common phrases, but what do they mean?

In The Practice, you will from time to time experience what is known as compartment burn; this is when something burns you up. This occurs when over a long period of time you stuff frustration and anger into a compartment. The more energy you stuff into the compartment, the more resistance builds in it. This mental resistance produces physical heat known as compartment burn. When one of these compartments is directed at another with consequence, you might hear someone say, "I just got burned."

Compartments that heat up are electrochemical thought-form images that can actually raise the temperature of the physical body. This is absolute proof of the connection between mind and body.

Keep in mind there are two spectrums of thought energy: disharmonious energy and harmonious energy. Disharmonious energy is from compartments, and harmonious energy is from your spirit. When compartments are dissolved, your spirit's harmonious energy appears in its place.

Where would you rather be—burnt-up in a compartment or cool, calm and collected in your spirit? Who really wants to be putting out fires all of the time?

As you do The Practice, you will begin to find and put out the fire from compartments.

When compartments engage you,
it's never
an enjoyable engagement.

Compartments in the Kelee —————→
feed by engaging

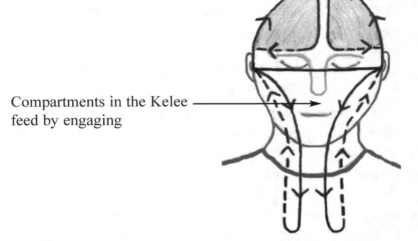

There are two basic ways compartments stay alive: by engaging you and by engaging others.

Compartments appear to have a mind of their own but they're not your conscious awareness. They do not have an electrochemical energy source of their own from the brain. Compartments are misperceptions of the mind masquerading as living entities; they do not have a viable energy source of their own, so they must take energy from others.

Compartments get energy by engaging your conscious awareness or someone else's. A compartment's first choice is usually another. Who wants to use their own energy when you can use someone else's? Have you ever been around someone who demanded your attention and you found yourself totally drained by your experience with him or her? This person fed from your energy, they literally sucked your energy. A common slang about such people is, "You suck!" There's another term for this kind of person, an energy vampire.

When compartments cannot feed from others, they are forced to feed from their own electrochemical energy source. This happens when a compartment makes you angry at yourself, when you whine, bitch or are just mad at the world in general. You create a negative environment in your mind that supports the compartments, which ironically ends up pulling from your immune system. Not good, eh?

You stop engaging compartments by not interacting with them, otherwise known as detachment in your mind.

If your mental attitude crashes,
so does your immune system.

Compartments draw energy ⟶
from the body 24/7

Our immune system is our first line of defense against disease. When it's working properly it's what keeps us healthy. The most important factor to keep your immune system at its optimum is your mental state. How you think and feel has a direct effect on your physical body.

The two major culprits in crashing your immune system are adrenaline and depression.

Adrenaline-based compartments pull massive amounts of energy from the physical body to produce a high, but are always followed by a huge crash. Adrenaline is by nature a fight or flight response best used for emergencies. It is not to be lived on or you will shorten your life span. Adrenaline-based compartments are also responsible for triggering adrenaline responses in others. Dealing with adrenaline compartments anywhere is draining! Dissolve the adrenaline compartments in you, and stay away from them in others. They will drain you.

Depressive-based compartments pull energy from you continuously. They are like black holes drawing energy in and depleting you at the same time. When you have a depression-based compartment fire, it's just a matter of time before you crash. It's no secret that when you are depressed you have no energy; it's hard to do anything, much less function to any degree of efficiency.

When you dissolve these compartments through The Practice, everything reverses. Energy starts appearing seemingly out of nowhere, actually; it's not being drained uselessly away. You'll be amazed when energy starts to flow how much stronger you feel.

*Your ideal life
is not of what's to come,
but what is ever present right now.*

When an ideal becomes ⟶
a compartment, it's not
an ideal situation

When you're seeking an ideal situation, it means you're looking for the world to fit your ideal of how you would like things to be. How often is everything in the world in its ideal place? A perfect situation is not waiting to please you. It's only important how pleased you are with yourself in any situation.

Ideals can be situations in the outside world or a thought-form image in your mind. If forceful energy is put into a thought-form image, it can compartmentalize into something that has a mind of its own. If a compartmentalized ideal is determining an outcome, you may not have a good outcome.

Idealized compartments don't have conscious awareness; they don't really know what they want. If an ideal drives you, it's your proof that a compartment is pushing you. There can only be one driver in your mind, you! The ideal state of mind is always when you are simply being yourself i.e., spirit, not an idealized compartment of yourself.

Remember when planning an ideal situation, there's a right time and a wrong time. Awareness will teach you the difference. The best time to plan something is when your mind is quiet and receptive. One clear thought of how to do something is worth more than a thousand scattered ideas.

Deeper than what ends up as a realized ideal is how you feel in each moment while you are attaining it. Isn't the ideal situation just your mind looking to feel good about yourself, right now?

*Worrying
about your life
is how you drain it from you.*

You worry about what you
do from your head

You worry about who you
are from your heart

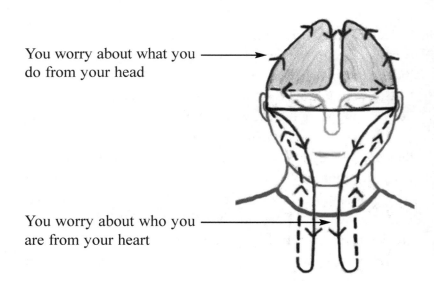

There are two basic kinds of worry: outside you and inside you.

1. **Worrying about what you do in the outside world.** This kind of worry is about what you have already done or what you're getting ready to do. This worry has already compartmentalized and is telling your conscious awareness something else is going to go wrong. The worrisome compartment feeds itself with potential fear to stay alive; it seems to have a mind of its own—the definition of a compartment.

When it comes to the outside world and worry—anticipation of the worst will find it. Thoughts are things; know what you set into motion before you do and you will worry less. The Practice will teach you how to see what you do, before you do it and teach you how to get rid of the worry from what you have already done. Big secret—if you clearly see, you don't worry.

2. **Worrying about who you are in your inside world.** Worries about who you really are, are all illusion and misperception! Common worries are: I'm ugly, I'm not accepted, I'm not loved, no one cares about me. Is there a good reason to feel bad about yourself? Maybe when you make a mistake, but when mistakes become lessons, worry ends. It is that simple.

File this away in big letters in your brain: *Everyone's spirit deep down is beautiful.* Everyone is heading toward the most beautiful place you could ever imagine. It's just a question of whether you know it or not. It's not living that takes all of the effort, it's worry.

There's nothing wrong with you,
other than
your own negative perception of you.

Unwarranted fears are
compartments that reside
in the Kelee

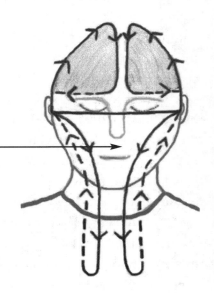

There are two basic kinds of fears: an unwarranted fear i.e., compartment, and a warranted fear i.e., the fight or flight response.

An unwarranted fear cannot physically hurt you but may make you believe it can. It is a compartment that can scare you. However, there is no real danger.

A warranted fear will trigger instinctual reaction and is a warning of real danger. This type of fear needs attention and may compartmentalize if your mind does not know how to deal with the threat properly.

When your conscious awareness cannot tell the difference between a compartment and bona fide fearing for your life, you will be forced to throw up a mental wall within your mind to protect yourself. You end up protecting yourself from a compartment within you. How safe can you feel living like this?

The only fears you're going to dissolve are your own. It will take doing The Practice over time to develop detachment, but I assure you, you can do it! When there is a space between you and your unwarranted fear, you'll know it's not you, only a negative influence casting a shadow on you.

All compartments are misperceptions. They're not real, but they can appear to be so. Remember, they're just states of mind that can appear as real, but are not the real you.

*If you're hiding behind walls,
you're hiding
from your own happiness.*

Walls are the block to your ⟶
happy experience of life

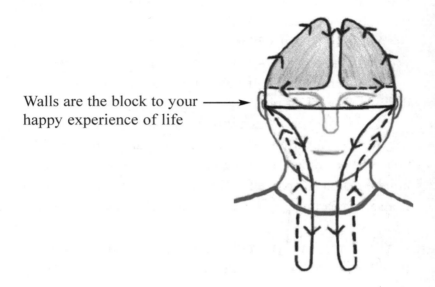

When you feel you must mentally protect yourself, the first response is to throw up a mental wall. To understand walls, you must first look to see if you're protecting yourself from another's negativity or if you're protecting yourself from being triggered because of your own negative compartments. If you sense the negative energy i.e., compartment, is coming from another person, you can just walk away. If the negative energy is in you, where can you go? If you feel negativity within you, are you protected from it and how?

If you have to protect yourself from yourself, you are imprisoned within your own mind. This fear-based wall feeds the compartment with fear to stay alive; you have made closed loop fear. Without knowing, the very thing you do not like about yourself—you keep alive.

When you live with the resistance of walls, they acclimate you to discontentment. When you still your mind through The Practice you'll drop your walls and stop feeding your compartments. You have now started the process of dissolving them, otherwise known as processing.

Walls do one thing well, they keep us from feeling good about ourselves. They do not protect us! If you're living with walls, they're blocking you from your own happiness. If you want to promote health and happiness, drop your walls and what you'll find is only you, standing there without them.

Emotional pain
is the misinterpretation
of what love really is.

Your head hurts because
you can't feel your heart

Your heart hurts because
you can't feel your spirit

Our head can take quite an emotional beating and put up with a lot of pain, but a deep heartache will take down the strongest of people.

If you're protecting yourself from feeling emotional pain, it means you're already in it, but don't want to look at it. When emotional pain compartmentalizes, it can totally consume you and make you do crazy things.

When love turns into emotional pain, it's because you tried to control your experience of love. The minute you start controlling love is the minute it stops being love. If love always precedes what you give, you will never hurt another. If you want to love another and your heart hurts, what you're giving comes from pain not love. Your heart is your opening to your spirit and can experience emotional pain or love. Remember, *emotional pain is the absence of love; emotional pain is not love! Love never hurts!*

As you open your heart to love, an inevitable realization dawns on you: that a loving nature is up to you, not someone else. It is sad that others may not be open to love, but alas, it is for each of us to find our way to our heart. Is not the way clear—the Kelee?

When your head is open to your heart and your heart is open to your spirit, all heartaches one day will disappear into the misinterpretation that they are. When your heart is open to love, emotional pain will heal; it is as simple as that.

*Anxiety is a compartment
that can't contain
its own negative energy.*

Anxiety is compressed
compartmentalized fear
in the Kelee

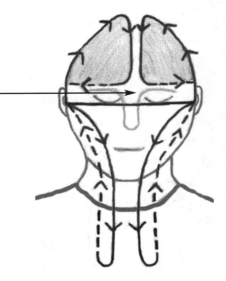

Everyone has felt anxiety at one time or another and it's one of the compartments that can totally consume you. Anxiety is formed when on a mental level you do not know how to deal with fear, so you stuff it! When you stuff fear, compartments become increasingly dense until electrochemically they spill over into the physical body as a reaction, which usually involves the shakes. Anxiety can be difficult to deal with in public places and is always awkward. Most people who have anxiety will generally not know what's causing it, because its energy is so strong. It overpowers the conscious awareness with a feeling of being totally out of control.

The Practice will dissolve anxiety, but it usually will take some time. After all, you have probably been stuffing your fear for a while. To help reverse anxiety, you must from your conscious awareness, stop stuffing what you fear and let The Practice do the rest. Imprint this on your brain, "If I feel anxiety, it's just a compartment, not me!"

What you need to know about yourself is most often what you don't. What you don't know about yourself can hurt you. This is why awareness is so important. How can you help yourself if you're in the dark about what's happening?

Anxiety is only a compartment and can be completely erased from your being. Do The Practice and anxiety will dissolve into the illusion of fear that it is!

When compartments
demand your attention,
you don't have any.

ADD is when multiple
compartments demand
attention at the same time →

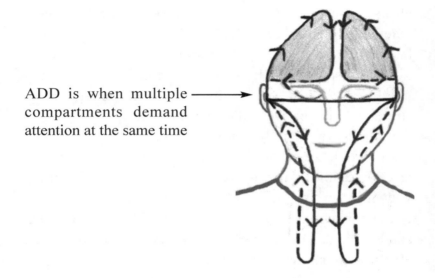

When your conscious awareness attaches to things and you cannot mentally let go of them, they compartmentalize in your Kelee. The compartments seem to have a mind of their own and many times all want attention at the same time. How can you do five things at once?

When you're hurrying to get things done you make mistakes, which means re-do's, which means wasted time; now you're starting to get frustrated. The faster you go the further behind you get as fragmentation escalates. In extreme cases this form of frustration can lead to hyperactive behavior.

You can only do so much within a given period of time and that's all; what you're really looking for is efficiency, not speed. Try this: pick up something in front of you, right now as fast as you can. Now put it down. Now pick up the same object, but calmly. What's the difference in time?

Did you notice the time to do each was only a fraction of a second apart? So why hurry? On a conscious level you can see what an illusion going fast is. Remember this exercise, consciously slow down and be mindful of what you're doing. If you're not, are you living?

The deeper problem with ADD is from multiple compartments associated with attachments and a need to do. As you dissolve the compartments through The Practice, your comprehension and efficiency will speed up. I have watched ADD disappear in many people, and if it's a problem with you, it will change. ADD is not a disease, it's a dysfunction.

Dissolve the distracting compartments and ADD will disappear. It's as simple as that.

*If you can't sleep at night,
you won't be awake by day.*

Compartments are the
number one reason you
can't sleep

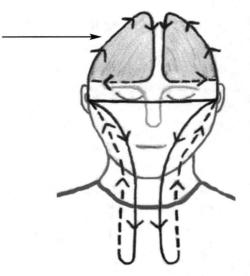

When you cannot get a good night's sleep, it can be hard to wake up. The brain, like the body, needs exercise and rest to run properly. The main reason people can't sleep is attachments to things they cannot let go of in their brain. Here is something you can't do anything about and yet you keep thinking about it. How many times has this happened to you when you want to sleep?

These attachments—known as compartments—engage your conscious awareness and won't let you relax and fall asleep. Whenever you think you must control people or things in the world, they have a hold on you, not you on them. Remember, *that which you hold onto, you must carry.*

Why can't you let go? Your conscious awareness does not know how to detach from brain function and the malfunction of compartments. It's that simple or hard, depending if you can detach or not.

The brain is just an organic computer. If it's running on autopilot who's in control? The Practice is like running a defrag program for your brain. It cleans out compartments weighing on your mind and organizes the brain for efficiency and optimum performance.

Sleep is care for you at night; The Practice is care for you in the daytime.

Remember, it's a peaceful mind that promotes peaceful sleep.

*There isn't a good reason
to be in a bad mood.*

PMS is just another name
for firing compartments in
the Kelee

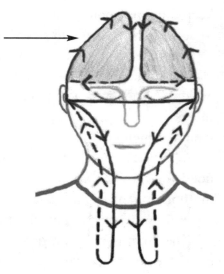

When your body requires more energy than usual to function, the energy has to come from somewhere. In the case of PMS, a woman cannot operate bodily function and hold up her mental walls at the same time. There is not enough electrochemical energy to run both.

When you cannot hold your walls up because of this lack of energy, you have no protection from your compartments and your conscious awareness is overwhelmed with negative emotion; irrationality and irritation have now taken control. This is not only a problem for women, but for the men who must endure its wrath and the trouble it causes in relationships.

The emotional effects of PMS can disappear in women, and I have observed it through The Practice. It's amazing when you're not irritated yourself, you don't irritate others. Men, you're gonna love this! As you do The Practice and your compartments disappear, the effects of PMS disappear. How much do you think solving this problem alone is worth to humanity?

Imagine if PMS was a non-issue in your life and you could have twenty-five percent more time in a month; wouldn't you rather be doing other things with your time?

Remember, *how you treat everyone matters.* You are always responsible for your actions, even at that time of the month. PMS isn't a disease, it's a dysfunction from compartments. When compartments go, so will PMS.

*Drugs
can dull the mask of negative emotion,
but only your spirit
can take the mask off.*

The real mask in life is a
misperception of oneself

When it comes to dealing with psychological emotional pain, drugs mask pain at best. Drugs can help in extreme cases to dull emotion, but it's never a long term solution. Recreational drugs used to escape emotional pain only make reality worse. The price you pay for what you get is too high and never worth the long-term side effects.

Drugs are unstable, with ups and downs, and there's still nothing stopping you from being consumed by a negative compartment while you're on them. Have you ever heard of a bad trip? Issues associated with drugs are actually spiritual ones; the deeper problem is always missing spiritual puzzle pieces.

It is true that negative emotions can alter our brain chemistry and cause other problems, but if the compartments causing the problem are dissolved, our chemistry normalizes naturally. The only stable, long lasting way to feel good is to eliminate the negative compartments causing your pain and learn to open to your spirit's well being.

The side effects of The Practice are all benefits. This may be hard to believe but true. Emotional pain needs to be healed by the spirit, not by drugs. When your conscious awareness is open to your spirit, it can open the body's natural healing ability to soothe your soul. Everything we need to feel good is within our reach, if we open our awareness to find it.

Emotional pain is a misperception of you, that's all.

*The extreme of a high
is often the prelude
to the crash of a low.*

Adrenaline and depression
compartments can appear
as bipolar

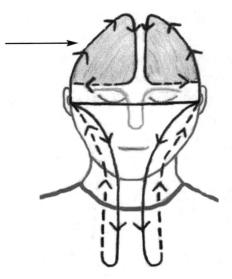

When it comes to bipolar disorder, it must be looked at carefully to see if it's a medical condition or a psychological one. If there's something wrong with the brain and it's not producing the right chemicals for healthy functioning, then it will need to be corrected with medication. If the problem is a psychological condition, then it can be corrected through The Practice, by dissolving the adrenaline and depression-based compartments.

If compartments have more strength than your conscious awareness and they're activated, they will consume you. When an adrenaline-based compartment is activated, it burns massive amounts of energy. When it runs out of energy, you default into a depression-based compartment, which then consumes you. You have just experienced being bipolar, but are you?

A supposed bipolar condition will disappear when the compartments associated with it disappear. If someone has been psychologically bipolar for a long time, their brain chemistry can change. However, this can be reversed through The Practice with healthy chemical function returning. We have an amazing ability to heal as a human, if we know how to help ourselves.

When a psychological bipolar condition is reversed through The Practice, it is an absolute miracle to observe. The Practice can make major changes in this area of the mind, and this is no theory!

Self-created realities
are mental breakdowns
waiting to happen.

Self-created realities are
compartments masquerading
as reality

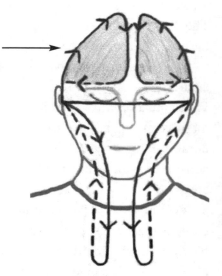

There are two kinds of mental breakdowns: medical and psychological. If a breakdown has to do with a physical problem in the brain, you had better see a doctor. When a mental breakdown is psychological, it's all in your head. The mind i.e., spirit, cannot break down. It's only an illusion that it can. A self-created reality is an illusion that your conscious awareness has built to escape compartments within your Kelee. If you have to create a positive attitude to offset a negative attitude, you're playing a game in your mind.

Electrochemically generated self-created positive attitudes must be fed energy. A self-created reality requires massive amounts of energy to sustain itself. And for what, something that's blocking you from the real experience of life?

Life is always wonderful on its own without you controlling it. When you're living in self-created realities, even if they're positive, you'll always feel they won't last. They can't, they're not real.

The breakdown you're looking for is of your compartments, not a self-created escape from them. When you do The Practice, you will set into motion the breakdown of compartments when you're at your strongest, not your weakest. The Practice teaches detachment from compartments, not separation from reality. Start The Practice so you can begin gaining mental strength today, while dissolving mental weakness at the same time.

The boogeyman
is only as real
as your thoughts or compartments
make him.

You cannot hide from a
worrisome compartment
when it's in you

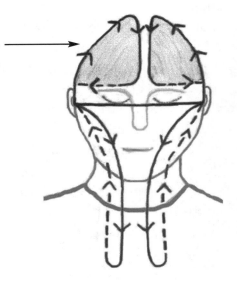

Compartmentalized fear occurs in three basic ways: manic fears, depressive fears and self-created escape from reality fears.

A lesser version of a self-created escape from reality is: fear of fear. There are actually times when people will create a scary scenario to distract them from a fear that's being triggered in them. This fear-based illusionary form of protection creates worry in your mind and keeps scary images alive. Worrying about what scares you will not control the outside world.

Fear of fear is actually your own worry and does not allow you to feel safe in life. A worrisome fear will not protect you from what may or may not happen. It's ironic that if you're already afraid, how are you keeping yourself safe? There's already fear within your conscious awareness, preceding what you're afraid to look at.

It takes massive amounts of energy to sustain worry, energy that would be better used for other things. Fear of fear is actually a fear of facing what scares you. How do you not face your life? You're already in it.

As you do The Practice you will drop this fear-based illusion of protection and realize what you have been doing to yourself all along. Detachment in your mind will replace fear of fear compartments and you will free yourself from this self-delusion for the last time.

Isn't it time for all of your boogeymen to become figments of past imagination, not reality?

> *When you live
> through programs,
> you do so
> at the expense of your life.*

Pervasive programs can
cover both hemispheres
of your brain

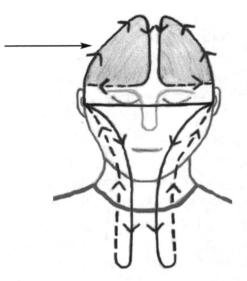

Pervasive programs are compartments so complete they can operate almost independent of mind function. It's widely known that through socialization you can pick up baggage. Just look around the world, notice any baggage in people?

Becoming a mold of how society thinks you should be is always at the expense of you living your life. There's an old saying, "When in Rome, do as the Romans do, or leave Rome." What if you live in Rome but don't feel Roman? How can you be yourself and at the same time fit into the outside world?

Fit into yourself, and you'll fit in anywhere!

How many times has your head gotten in your way? You thought one thing but did another. How does this happen? You can't be conscious of what you're doing, if you're living through a pervasive compartment. You become as the expression goes, "A head case."

To have true self-expression, you must fit into your own mind i.e., spirit, not into the outside world. A wise man once said, *"Be in the world but not of it."* Your spirit can do this because it has a presence but no mass. Your spirit is in the world but not physically of it. Your mind i.e., spirit, can live anywhere, except in programs! Programs are not really you or reality.

As your conscious awareness lives more in your mind i.e., spirit, you will spot these elusive programs and free yourself from society's illusion of living, once and for all.

When you touch to take,
you abuse.

A compartment in your
head is a block to touch

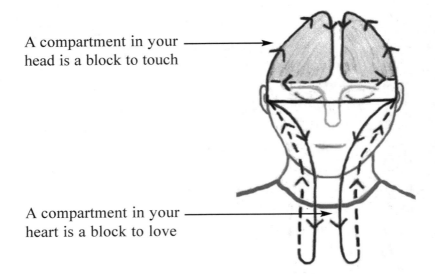

A compartment in your
heart is a block to love

When a destitute soul takes without regard for another, the consequence can be disastrous. It is one of the deepest violations of the soul there is. Sexual abuse is not an easy area to look at in the mind, but if you're blocking out this darkness, you may have to live with it for the rest of your life. You don't have to!

If someone is sexually abused, it compartmentalizes either in the lesser or greater Kelee with the abused individual probably abusing someone else. The abusive compartment may try to convince the conscious awareness that the behavior is appropriate. If the abusive compartment succeeds, the person abusing will not think they have a problem. The compartment is stronger than their conscious awareness, so the abuse continues.

If sexual abuse compartmentalizes in the greater Kelee, the abused person may think it's their fault and bury or shut off their healthy sexual feelings. Buried sexual frustration can cause relationship problems and even worse, cause long-term confusion with the abused not knowing right from wrong.

Through The Practice, you can dissolve any sexual abuse compartment and learn to live free from the harmful effects of past unfortunate circumstances. Remember, *every compartment that's installed can be dissolved.*

If you've been abused in any way, know there's a way out of the pain, into the healing space of your spirit found in the Kelee.

The void of emptiness starts
when fulfillment in life stops.

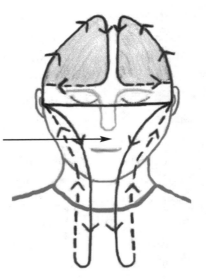

If you're full of compartments,
you're empty of life

In actuality, there are two forms of emptiness: compartments that are empty of life and your mind i.e., spirit, that is empty of compartments.

Everyone at some time has felt empty inside; if you mentally close down to life, you will open to the void of emptiness. You end up in the void when you do not know how to open up to your mind i.e., spirit. If you feel empty of life, it's because you can't feel. If you want to experience fulfillment in life, you must learn to feel from your spirit.

The way out of the void is understood when you learn what stops fulfillment from entering the Kelee. The entry is blocked by the energy of compartments pushing out in an attempt to take life in. When you need to take in life, you never receive from it. The proverbial void of emptiness forms when the Kelee is filled with negative compartments; these compartments draw energy in and give grief out. Compartments never open you to experience, they take the experience of life away.

Compartments are predetermined thought-form images deciding how they experience life, that's why they don't experience it. To open up, you must realize why the void of destitution from compartments is closing you down.

It's up to each individual to understand and maintain his or her own mind. If you're ignorant, you may end up living in the void of compartments. If you're aware, you'll end up in the fulfillment of your spirit. The choice is yours.

When you know you're lost
is when
you really start looking.

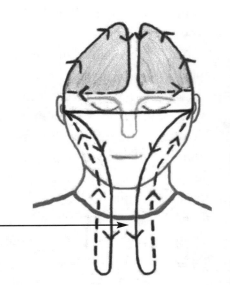

When you cannot feel —
your heart, you are lost
in your own soul

The greatest motivating factor on the planet is pain. Pain will eventually drive everyone to self-understanding. If not, suffering will continue until you realize what's causing the pain and learn the spiritual lessons to end it. Deeper than what you do is, specifically within your mind, why you do what you do. This brings you to learn about the deeper workings of your mind, understanding your conscious awareness, compartments, the Kelee and your spirit.

Destitution happens when you're unaware of your own mind and when something you don't understand drives your life into painful situation after painful situation. Destitution occurs when your spirit cannot open to life because of compartments. Destitution is always associated with negativity and so this is where everyone must begin to troubleshoot their mind. Negative feelings always come from misperceptions of life.

If you are to feel good about yourself, you must first understand why you do not. A destitute feeling is like being homeless within your own soul. As simple as it can be said, destitution is the absence of feeling love; it's a disconnection from your spirit.

No one's soul is really destitute, just misunderstood. Have no fear, the miracle to end destitution is here and within your own mind the ability to bring about change.

When you never lose sight that your love comes from within, you will never be lost in your own soul ever again.

*Grace is the absence
of bullcrap!*

Bullcrap is when someone
is full of compartments in
the Kelee

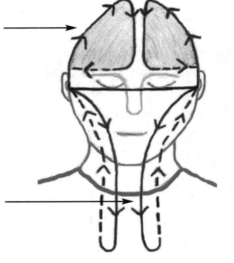

Grace is when someone
lives free from bullcrap in
the Kelee

When we talk about being in a state of grace, it is usually thought to be some exalted spiritual state of being associated with a priest or the clergy.

Who decides who's in a state of grace and who's not? If bullcrap comes out of your mouth, didn't you decide where you are? Truly, grace can be described in two ways: the absence of bullcrap or the true nature of your spirit.

It will be a fine day when it is commonplace to openly call someone on their crap i.e., compartments, and not get into an argument on whether it stinks or not. How many times have you heard someone say, "If that isn't a load of bull," or "You're full of crap." Bullcrappy feelings will end when they're no longer in you, as compartments. It has been said, "Everyone wants to get to heaven, but nobody wants to walk through crap to get there." The only good crap is the crap you have gotten rid of yourself—namely compartments —and this will happen through The Practice.

When it comes to being in a state of grace, it is a state of awareness in your spirit. Have you not noticed that whenever someone is graceful, it is always beautiful? Is this not where you want to be?

Open to your greater Kelee and you will realize a state of grace that kings and queens wished they had. Yet, it is there for everyone, if you know where to find it.

*The outside world
adds to life
but does not
give it.*

Chapter Five

The Lesser Kelee

All the struggle in life
is to find
what you already have,
the freedom
to live your own life.

*We find the greater in us
by understanding
the lesser first.*

The lesser Kelee is where brain
and mind i.e., spirit, meet

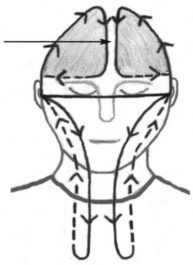

If you look closely at the Kelee diagram, you'll notice that the greater and lesser Kelee are actually one Kelee folding in upon itself. The Kelee is the containment field and interface between your physical nature and your spiritual nature. The Kelee brings us together as a unified being. The energy of the lesser Kelee extends from the surface of the mind, moves up, around and in between both hemispheres of the brain, where it folds into the brain network. The lesser Kelee is where brain function meets mind function i.e., spirit, with your conscious awareness determining how aware you are of your spirit in the Kelee—lesser and greater.

The brain is often referred to as the small mind because it lacks the wisdom of the spirit. Your brain uses a thinking process to deduce and likes to be in control, even when what you are about to do feels wrong. This gut level feeling is commonly called a conscience in the lesser aware state and called knowing in the greater aware state.

When you begin the first part of The Practice and your conscious awareness is in the lesser Kelee area, it is quite difficult to be detached from the controlling brain network and heavy compartmentalization you will first encounter in your head. However, with time as you do The Practice, you can actually be in your head, without being out of your mind.

Data isn't a definition
of who you are.
How wisely your mind uses data is.

The intellect i.e., brain, is ⟶
basically an organic computer

The intellect is marvelous by nature. It receives, analyzes, sorts and stores information. Think of your brain as the hard drive of a computer, with the surface of your mind being the RAM—random access memory—and your spirit as the user. Your computer is only as good as your mind i.e., spirit's ability to run it.

Many times out of fear, people will superimpose information over the brain in an effort to not forget something. However, what ends up happening is clutter begins to build up, otherwise known as compartments. This clutter ends up slowing down the brain's efficiency and creates unneeded distractions. If you start operating through these compartments and stop using the memory of your brain, the pathways in the brain may start closing down. If you're not careful, compartments can crash operations, unless these destructive programs are deleted. Think of compartments in your Kelee as computer viruses that constantly interfere with daily performance.

Any part of your brain that you don't use will start to shut down. Memory is an important part of any computer, organic or not. As you begin doing The Practice and compartments break down, your mind will clean up as your memory improves. Think of The Practice as a defragmentation program for your mind.

When your spirit directs electrochemical energy through a well-running intellect, you can do amazing things.

Food for thought
is more literal
than you may think.

Harmonious thoughts promote
energy, negative thoughts
deplete it

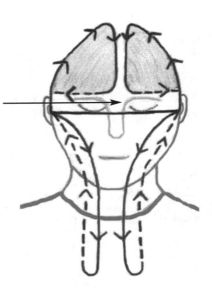

Electrochemical energy is the energy of the physical self; it's the energy that sustains our physical body and the brain network. When our electrochemical energy quits, we call it death.

As your conscious awareness becomes in tune through The Practice, you will realize that the law of moderation rules electrochemical energy. If you push past moderation, detriment happens. This is an absolute! Yes it's true, when you're young you can "burn the candle at both ends," however, if you look back, you always paid your dues in suffering. Nevertheless, why subject yourself to this detriment?

If you want your thought process to be clear, your electrochemical energy must be stable. As you begin to work with moderation in your energy level, your conscious awareness calms down and the deeper awareness of mind function begins to emerge. As this long term shift from brain function to mind function happens, another amazing phenomenon occurs—you don't crash anymore. Your mind i.e., spirit, knows your brain's limitations and stops you before a crash.

Once your conscious awareness is stable, your mind will begin to realize the effects of thought and energy. Negative thoughts pull energy while harmonious thoughts promote energy. Understanding how the thought to energy equation in your mind works is an amazing learning process.

Right now, you can have no idea how far The Practice will take you. Your mind is what opens you to the ultimate experience in life, and there is no finer time to start than now.

*There's nothing you can do
about death except live every day
without the worry of it.*

Warranted fears are instinctual
fears triggered by the brain

There seems to be great confusion in people about what a warranted fear is and what an unwarranted fear is. When it comes to warranted fear, it's triggered instinctually when we need the fight or flight response for an emergency.

Warranted fears are here to protect us, not to threaten us.

For many people, the fear of death from the brain is very real, because the brain can die and it knows it. Not much is preordained but one thing is for sure, one day our body will cease to function. If you are not living a fulfilled life and come to the end of it, you will feel the void of emptiness associated with destitution. Can you think of a worse thought than to come to the end of your life, look back and feel, "My life meant nothing!"?

The real fear associated with the fear of death is that you did not really live. If you're not open to your spirit, you may feel like the walking dead right now. The reason people commit suicide is they already feel dead, so why continue to live? The main reason you won't feel alive is due to compartments living from the past; they're blocks to living in the present. When you live from your spirit, you can't die; it's non-physical. This is why the spirit is referred to as having everlasting life.

Do The Practice and I can assure you, you will not come to the end of your life with regret but with a light heart, looking forward to the next adventure.

Awareness is the ultimate
form of self-protection.

Self-preservation is instinctual
protection from the brain

Self-awareness is protection
from your spirit

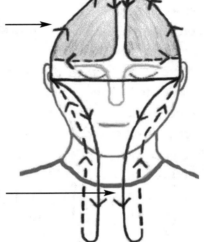

There are two basic forms of self-protection: fear-based self-preservation from the brain and self-awareness from your spirit. Self-preservation is instinctual from the brain and automatic if you need it.

Self-awareness protection from your spirit is learned. When you can learn to read vibrations and can sense potential trouble before it gets to you, you can move in a different direction. Truly, even a martial arts master knows the best fight is no fight at all. No matter how good you can be, someone else can be better. One error in a fight can result in lifelong suffering. It is much wiser to not be in situations where your life is in danger.

When you're walking through life, walk with your awareness wide open, if you sense potential harm coming your way, simply walk a different direction. Some might say this is paranoia. There's a big difference between awareness and paranoia; awareness operates without fear, paranoia operates in fear.

As you do The Practice, your ability to sense what is around you will open naturally as you start using your conscious awareness. Knowing the range of vibrations from disharmony to harmony will not only open your spiritual eyes to potential harm, but also to the beauty of life. It is always a good practice to be mindful in life, whether you are protecting yourself or not.

Adrenaline is a high
but always
at the expense of a low.

Adrenaline is the small mind's ⟶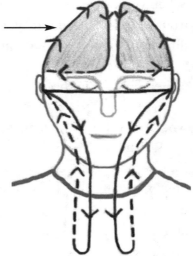
drug of choice

Adrenaline is an instinctual fight or flight response in the brain and a powerful drug that produces an enormous high, but at an expense.

Everyone will experience adrenaline from time to time, but it's not wise to live on it. It's a coarse form of energy and difficult to control with one major drawback: every time adrenaline is triggered, it's always followed by a crash. This is the big mood swing people experience when living on it. It feels great to be up, but the down is really a downer.

Adrenaline can be triggered through the instinctual process of your brain or it can be triggered by a compartment within your mind. If you're triggering adrenaline by your activities, know you may be in a dangerous situation. It's not for anyone else to say what another should do with his or her lifestyle, but it is good to be aware of what you're getting into before you do. Keep in mind that adrenaline is also associated with the manic side of manic-depressive disorders and if you're not careful, you can cross the line. Hence, the expression, "I've gone too far!"

It would be wise to know that adrenaline keeps you in your small mind by the nature of the energy itself. Is this where you want to live?

Remember, adrenaline will shorten your life if you live on it. It is by nature a short-term high. However, know there is another way to live, from the long-term vibrant energy of your spirit. Weigh carefully everything you do in life; it's called contemplation, the way of wisdom.

Attachment to things
is a headache.

The brain attaches, it lives in a
3-D world, it likes to control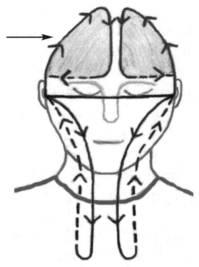

Whenever you try to control life, whether it is people or things, you form mental attachments. These mental attachments become compartmentalized in your Kelee. What appears to be bothering you outside with attachments is actually bothering you inside from compartments.

The brain lives in the world of sense-consciousness or the three-dimensional world, and relies on the physical senses to bring us experience. It's easy to see why we attach to things, if what we mentally touch is harmonious, our sense of touch gives us a feeling of being connected and accepted. However, if we cannot let go of what we touch, even if it feels good, attachments form ultimately causing pain.

If what we touch is negative and we can't let go, a negative compartment forms in our Kelee and now starts affecting us. When attachments form in the lesser Kelee, they can electrochemically compartmentalize and give us headaches —literally and physically—if the energy is concentrated enough. How often have you been in a situation and thought to yourself, "This is such a headache?" If you're not careful, it will become a real one in your head. In the brain network, compartments can form tension headaches that can range from mild to migraine. In fact, most headaches are caused from compartments.

If you want to free your mind of headaches, free your mind of compartments. You'll be amazed at how much better it is to use meditation i.e., The Practice, instead of medication to free your mind from this pain.

When baggage
becomes your furniture,
you become uncomfortable
in your own home.

Baggage in the lesser Kelee
has to do with what we think
we need

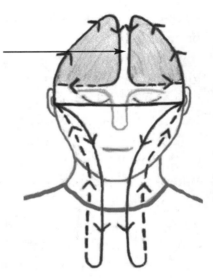

As you begin doing The Practice and start opening your spiritual eyes, you will begin to sense compartments. Your mind sees in what is known as thought-form images. When you think of an apple, it is not A-P-P-L-E. You think of what an apple looks like.

When compartments form from the negative circumstances of life, they take the shape of how you experienced them. This can include visual images, sounds, smells, touch and even taste. They are little worlds of their own that can control you whether you're aware of them or not.

Baggage in the lesser Kelee area has to do with how you feel about the outside world. The images that form in the lesser Kelee can look like: **cabinets:** places to hide parts of us, **chest of drawers:** secret things we hide about ourselves, **bookshelves:** information we don't want to forget—we might look stupid, **moving boxes:** have to do with how you store information that you don't know what to do with. All of these images are superimposed over the brain so as not to be forgotten. I have seen images of **brooms:** cleaning issues, **rugs:** trying to feel at home, **lots of furniture:** classic baggage—I need this, **suitcases:** needing to always be on the move.

When baggage has become your furniture, you carry it around as weight in and on your mind. Baggage simply interferes with how you operate in your life. How would you like to drop it for the last time? Remember, *what you mentally hold onto, you must carry.*

When you create reality,
life stops being real.

True reality is perceived ——
from clarity in the Kelee

When you cannot face the hardship of reality, you most likely will change it to fit what you are comfortable with. I say hardship because if reality is beautiful, you do not have to change it. In actuality, we as humans don't create reality, we perceive it as it is. We only need to self-create an escape from our life when it's not good enough.

Everything you do is a thought before it's a manifestation of something. If your reality is a mess, you'll have to decide if you created the mess or it's a mess of its own accord. If you created the mess, why did you do it? If you're being directed by a negative compartment, then what manifests will be negative. If you're seeing through a compartment, you're seeing through a negative filter. If you're not receiving information clearly, how can you make clear decisions?

As compartments dissolve through The Practice, your mind i.e., spirit, will have a clear space in the compartment's place. The space of your spirit is freedom and always feels good. If you feel good before you do something, everything can only get better. Haven't you ever noticed that when your heart feels good, reality is always beautiful?

When the world is a mess on its own and you want to help clean it up, don't you need to have clarity to know how to do it, not just good intentions? Clarity is what happens as a by-product of The Practice.

When your spiritual eyes open, they see clearly.

Reality is what it is. What makes reality heaven or hell is what comes from within us. If you want to be real, clean up what isn't.

Passion is a drive to do,
but by who
or what?

Passion is a need to fulfill
what you feel is missing
in your spirit

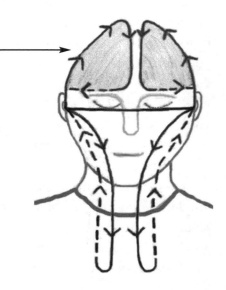

Passion manifests in two basic ways: through things and/or people.

When you're passionate about things, you'll notice you're always driven to do what you do. However, where is this drive coming from? The drive is a need to fulfill you in some way. This drive can get things done, but how are you feeling while being driven, tormented or contented?

When it comes to passionate relationships, you'll notice that they're the most exciting and the most painful at the same time. When you're passionate about someone, there's always a need to get from them. If you're passionate about another and they feel the same way as you, it's euphoric. If not, it's extremely painful. Passion forms attachments, which causes a need to control, which produces jealousy and suffering. Passionate behavior is the physical response to fulfill what we don't feel from our spirit.

Remember, this is your life to live and if you feel the need to explore passion, do so; you may need to learn something. It's interesting to note, passion is quite often associated with the phrase, "I don't know what drove me to do it?"

Watch where the energy of passion comes from and you'll find it's coming from some place other than you. This other place would be wise to explore. Your spirit is never driven by some unknown source. It's always brain function and the malfunction of compartments that push you. When you get in touch with the depths of your spirit, you'll find it does long to complete itself but does not forcibly push you to do so.

Domination is a temporary illusion
at best.

When your head has to be
in control, your spirit is not

One of the biggest problems in the world is people trying to dominate others. Collectively mankind will have to get together and decide what to do.

The answer to finding peace is simple; it's called the spiritual law of harmony, non-interference. For those who continue operating in ignorance of this spiritual law, a heavy price will be paid. Mentally controlling another is the lesser form of what we call slavery and is simply wrong!

Along with domination is always mental intimidation. If you have to have it only your way, others are always excluded, causing discontentment. Have you ever heard the expression, "Someone has a big head?" Actually, shouldn't it be, "What a small mind?" When you need to be more than who you are, you have just made yourself less.

When you don't have to prove your point, you can be open to understanding another's.

When you're open to how your mind sees, you can learn to read negative thought-form images. Negative energy always spirals downward! This negativity is of course from compartments, the root of all disharmony on the planet. People who try to dominate another's life are always out of control themselves. Sadly enough, if they lead, they lead people into suffering.

Look at the drawing of the greater Kelee, now feel your heart in this place. Can you actually convince yourself from your heart that controlling another is right?

When everyone looks into their own heart and stops hurting themselves, we as people will stop hurting each other. It is as simple as that!

*Morals are intellectual religious laws
enforced from your head.
Wisdom is governed by spiritual laws
from your heart.*

Morals are religious laws
written for your head

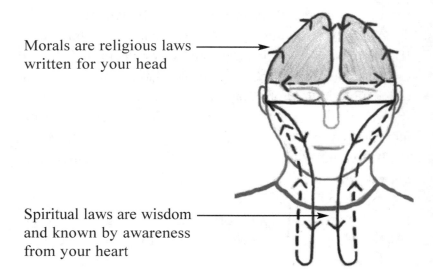

Spiritual laws are wisdom
and known by awareness
from your heart

Morals are basic guidelines for people who can't control their actions, much like civil laws but much more difficult to enforce. Guilt is usually how moral laws are enforced; however, guilt only makes you feel worse and doesn't solve problems.

If everyone followed morals, we wouldn't have any crimes and yet how often do people justify immoral acts from their head? Truly, if you live from your heart i.e., spirit, you will make your wisest decisions in life. If you do make a mistake, learn from it and don't do it again. Remember, you're not perfect but that doesn't mean you are hopelessly flawed. You're on an adventure of a lifetime to find your spiritual puzzle pieces.

When you have the awareness to know why you make hurtful mistakes, you will stop making them!

When you start living from your spirit instead of your head, you begin to feel more lighthearted with each passing day. When you don't need an ego and don't have negative compartments controlling you, your spirit will open to the freedom life has to offer, and then morals and civil laws will cease to be broken.

Remember, when you follow the spiritual laws of right and wrong found in your heart, you will not have to live under the weight of a moral structure ever again. Trust your heart i.e., spirit. It really does know the way out of all trouble.

When you open to your heart and your heart opens to your spirit, freedom opens to you.

*Time
is your experience of it.
Happy or sad,
it's up to you.*

Linear time is experienced from ⟶
the brain in three dimensions

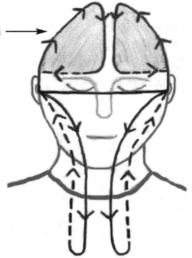

Linear time is measured as matter moving through space and there's not much we can do about changing it. It's associated with the three-dimensional space of height, width and depth. We work within these planes of awareness associated with the lesser Kelee to understand the world in which we live.

Linear time is constant and keeps coming, whether we like it or not. It would be wise to like it. If you're worrying about time, you're not living. If you're truly living life, you'll embrace time and enjoy living. If you're not comfortable with time, why don't you ask yourself why?

You'll be comfortable with time when time isn't a concern—in other words—when you're not worrying about time from your head! When you're living from your mind i.e., spirit, instead of the chronological time of your brain, you'll feel like a happy-go-lucky kid again. A wise man once said, "To enter the kingdom of heaven you must become as a small child."

If you're not celebrating life each day, what reason do you have for even being born?

Have you not noticed, *true happiness is experienced in the birth of each moment?*

The golden moments of life are up to us to experience. If we love life, it feels like heaven, if we do not, it feels like hell. When you do The Practice long enough and get out of your measuring brain and into your mind i.e., spirit, you'll find that time is our creation of it. What we do with it, happy or sad is our experience of time, determined by our wise use of it.

*What you see
outside yourself
is always preceded
by how you see
inside yourself.*

Chapter Six

The Greater Kelee

*Wisdom is always understood
individually
before it's understood
collectively.*

Finding your spirit
takes nothing more
than knowing where to look.

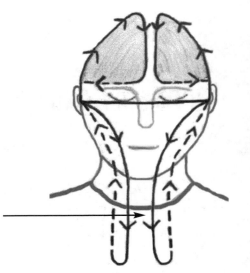

This is where your spirit
is centered

Everyone has had the sensation of having emotion welling up from within them but few people have ever stopped and asked why. This emotion wells up from a phenomenon known as the greater Kelee. Kelee (pronounced "key-lee") is an ancient *Sanskrit* word meaning, *having to do with different states of mind.* The phenomenon of the Kelee is a field of energy that drops from the surface of the mind, down inside to about where your heart is. Then it turns upward flowing around and down in between both hemispheres of the brain to form the lesser Kelee.

There's a famous saying, *the eyes are the windows to the soul.* Guess what you're looking into when you look into someone's eyes and feel depth in them? The opening of the greater Kelee is literally the entrance to your heart and soul. The greater Kelee is where your spirit is centered. That's why, when you feel love, you feel your heart—not your physical heart—your spiritual one. As you do The Practice and spend time in your greater Kelee, you will experience this as the truth.

As you do The Practice and explore your Kelee, you will unlock the mystery of your mind. Everything you understand is understood through your mind i.e., spirit. The greater Kelee is where your spirit resides and where all problems are solved. All saints and sages throughout time have said to go to this place and yes, what you are looking for, really is within you.

*Find the space
that's you,
and you'll find your spirit.*

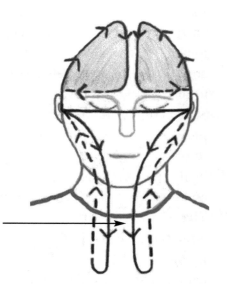

You connect to your spirit
by dropping your conscious
awareness here

To connect to your spirit, you must first know how and where to find it. The two biggest blocks to finding your spirit are ego and compartments.

When you create an ego, it's because you cannot feel your spirit. This self-creation of you compartmentalizes your conscious awareness as a separate, non-feeling entity. This non-feeling state of mind feels devoid of life and out of touch with reality.

Individual compartments are the next block to your spirit because they think they have a mind of their own. However, you can only have one mind or it's insanity and yet each compartment seems to have a mind of its own.

Everyone's brain is filled with compartmentalized tension. Feel yours right now and you'll know it's true. The first step of The Practice associated with the lesser Kelee will begin to relax your tension-based mind. As you begin to let go and dissolve tension associated with the lesser Kelee area, you'll drop into the greater Kelee where your spirit is centered. Your spirit will appear as empty space but it's not empty, it's non-physical. Whenever you need your own space, this is where you need to be, connected to your spirit. The emptiness in your spirit is actually the opening to fulfillment, not the empty feeling associated with destitution.

If you want to connect to your spirit, here is the way: drop your conscious awareness into your greater Kelee, be still and your spirit will come to you.

When you don't have space within,
you don't have space anywhere.

The lesser Kelee space ——————

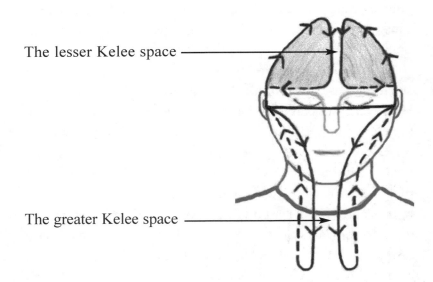

The greater Kelee space ——————

It is quite common to hear people say, "I need some space!" Most often when someone says this, what they really mean is, "I want you out of my space." This is usually when someone is imposing his or her thoughts on another. A wise teacher once said to me, "It's amazing, when you don't do things to people, they like it!"

You can always walk away from someone imposing on your space, but what about your own compartments imposing on you? What if your Kelee is filled with compartments?

Compartments are the reason why it's hard to feel your spirit; they block access to it. Not only can your space be crowded with compartments but also with chatter from the brain infringing on your conscious awareness. When you don't crowd your mind with too many thoughts, you allow space to occur.

The space you're trying to find is within your Kelee. This space is where your spirit is found and the only place you really experience life.

As you do The Practice, overcrowding in your Kelee by compartments and excessive thoughts will simply change into open space and freedom. This uninterrupted space is called peace and is found in your Kelee.

If you don't have a quiet space in your mind, how can you be peaceful anywhere?

You find yourself
in yourself.

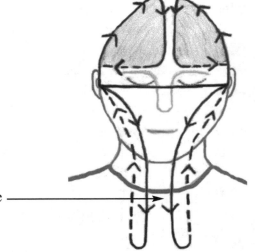

You find yourself here ——————————————→

To find who you are, you must know where to look. *You find yourself in yourself.* This phrase is so simple and yet so profound.

You are not your brain, it's an organic computer; it runs your physical body and stores data. You are not your issues or compartments; they're misperceptions of you. They're patterns formed by either your own self-creation, or another's view of you that you took on as your own.

You are your mind i.e., spirit; they are one and the same!

The pathway to enlightenment is understanding the difference between the delusion of misperception from compartments and the reality of clear perception from your mind i.e., spirit. You find clear perception by finding your spirit. Now, there is a way and here is the map. If you go inside yourself, in your greater Kelee, every day and still your mind, you will find clarity! It will take patience, but as you shift from brain function into mind function, you will start to see yourself like never before.

All masters throughout time have said to go within. One famous teacher said it very well, "Where your heart is, there also will you find your treasure." Your heart is the doorway to your spirit, with you being the only person who can decide to open the door or close it. If you turn away from your emotional pain, you close the door. If you face your emotional pain, you open the door.

If you want love in your life, don't you think your heart would be a good place to spend some time? This may be the most valuable piece of information you will ever read!

*Patience
isn't a measure of time,
it's a quality of living.*

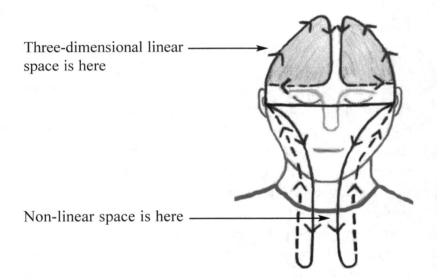

Three-dimensional linear space is here

Non-linear space is here

If you want to learn patience, you must get out of the three-dimensional space of the brain. How you do this is by living in your spirit. Your spirit lives by experiencing each moment, not by measuring them.

The biggest time-stealer in life is ego. An ego constantly strives excessively and never seems to get enough. This need to get will put your conscious awareness out of phase with your spirit and out of touch with reality. If your attention is always out ahead of you, you're never centered in the moment. This sets up a feeling of being uncomfortable with yourself, which can extend to others around you as an irritating vibration. If you irritate yourself, you will irritate others.

The second biggest time-stealer is compartments, which are worry-based time capsules trying to replicate previous experiences in time. The ironic thing about replicating compartments is you did not feel good when they formed and you won't when you relive them.

Patience is not something you can experience by deciding it from your head, but by living from your spirit, which has no linear mass to measure the passing minutes. When your conscious awareness is in your greater Kelee, you will begin to understand what being patient really is.

Time is what you experience from it. It's a quality of living, not a measure of time.

You will master the now
when you do not want
to leave it.

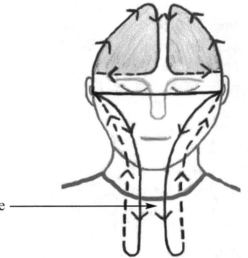

The now is found in the
space of your spirit

When you find yourself impatient, it means you don't like where you are right now. Looking to the future will not make you feel patient. If you're not in this moment, you're missing your life.

The key to being in "the now" is learning to live in your spirit. Your spirit does not know how to be impatient because it lives in non-linear space without time. Your spirit does not know how to be any other place other than where it is. All your spirit knows is how to experience life.

Space in your mind, otherwise known as the now, offers the luxury of being present and paying attention because you're not pushed. The now of your spirit can't be pushed; the future does not exist yet. When you live from your spirit you accept life uninterrupted. It's easy to pay attention because you're interested in what you're doing. Remember, the pathway to enlightenment is just another name for a self-interest study.

When you allow the experience of life to enter the surface of your mind, flow through the greater Kelee and into the lesser Kelee, you'll feel like you're living like never before. When you feel happy in your mind, you do not need to be someplace else and being in the now is achieved. Have you ever noticed, you never seem to hurry from a place you like to be?

Life's speed limit is being comfortable with the now. As if you can really live anyplace else.

You cannot be comfortable outside, until you're comfortable inside the space of your spirit.

Non-linear moments
are the beginning
of that
which has no ending.

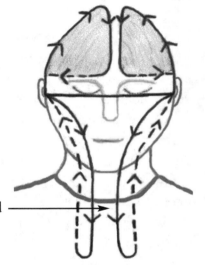

Non-linear time is experienced
in the space of your spirit

The non-linear space of your spirit is in a realm that has no matter, so there's no chronological time as we know it. How you understand the three-dimensional linear world is determined by how you perceive it from your non-linear mind i.e., spirit. Your physical senses bring you the linear world, however, it takes your spirit to understand it.

Why does everyone seem to perceive the world differently? It's because the understanding within our individual spirits are at different levels of self-knowledge and awareness.

The non-linear space of your spirit allows you to experience life without the hard constraints of three-dimensional reality. As the distractions of sense consciousness subside and compartments dissolve, you begin to have more time to yourself. This time in your mind will open you to self-understanding; it is as simple as that! It's amazing the freedom your conscious awareness can experience when it's in the greater Kelee free from analyzation.

The long-term goal of The Practice is to learn to live from the non-linear space of your spirit. Your spirit is called the big mind for good reason; it's the beginning of a way of comprehending that has no ending. Your spirit is the opening to a realization of infinity and a freedom in your mind you cannot imagine.

Remember, you learn from your mind by spending time with it. The mind ceases to be a mystery when you learn to see it for what it is. Open to the non-linear space of your spirit and you will open to the eternal moment.

Trust is the acceptance
of what you feel,
good and bad.

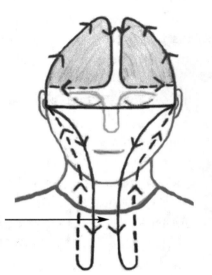

Trust is an acceptance of what
your spirit clearly perceives

Trusting in what your spirit perceives is one of the deepest experiences you will face in your life. If you cannot trust what you feel, you will be forced to question what trust is.

Trust ultimately will come down to your conscious awareness knowing what your heart feels. It's easy to trust a good feeling about yourself but hard to trust a bad feeling about yourself. This is a huge clue in understanding your heart. It's easy to trust a good feeling about yourself because that's who you really are. However, if a bad feeling comes up from within, your conscious awareness may think this negativity is actually you. This can be scary as hell! This negative feeling is just a compartment trying to convince you that you are someone other than who you really are.

The way to tell who you are and who you are not, is by moving your conscious awareness into mind function so you can clearly see the malfunction of compartments. There are only two things in your Kelee, your spirit and compartments. Your spirit is the real you, and compartments the negative misperception of you.

As you do The Practice and drop your conscious awareness into your greater Kelee, the day will come when you will have to let go and trust that you will not disappear into the space of your spirit.

It really is easy to trust, when you realize that when you let go of hell, heaven will appear.

When your heart feels heavy,
it's not your heart you feel,
it's baggage!

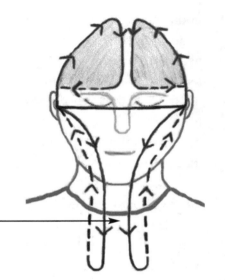

Baggage in the greater
Kelee has to do with
how you feel about you

The baggage i.e., compartments, in your greater Kelee are some of the most painful emotions you will ever experience. Compartments in the greater Kelee can be any image you can imagine; here are a few of the most agonizing ones.

A tar pit: total despair, these are of the deepest depression compartments. **A black hole:** a feeling of futility. **A dark space:** lesser in intensity than the first two but still intense emotional pain. **Mud:** feeling like you're stuck. **A person striking another:** an abuse issue. **Spires of energy:** controlling people telling you how you should be; on some level you have given up control to another and have lost yourself. **Trunks:** a place to hide secrets about yourself, feeling ashamed of yourself. Some compartments can be just feelings without images, like feeling downtrodden, left behind or feeling less than.

Every negative emotion about how you could feel bad about yourself will manifest in the greater Kelee. All compartments in the greater Kelee are all misperceptions of you. You have either bought someone else's negative view of you, or self-created a negative view of you, yourself.

When you sense a compartment influencing your conscious awareness, trust what you sense as being what it is! *Never forget, anything negative within you is not the real you!* Your true nature is not negative; it's a beautiful openness to life.

Ironically, *all the struggle is to find what we already have, a beautiful spirit.*

The only protection
you have from compartments
is the feeling of safety
when you don't have them.

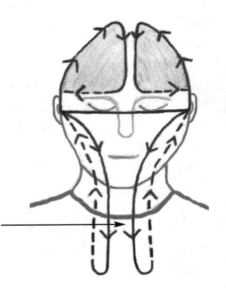

Compartments in the Kelee
appear as the illusion of
reality

Inward Self-protection

One of the grandest illusions in humanity is that you can protect yourself from feeling your own dysfunction. All you do is get comfortable with being uncomfortable.

Intellectually coping with an issue does not work; all this does is put a fear-based wall between you and your compartment. This fear-based wall inadvertently feeds the issue and makes a closed loop of dysfunction. The deeper fear in your conscious awareness is that the compartment might really be you or it might consume you and could become you.

The way you free yourself from your issues is by moving your conscious awareness into your mind i.e., spirit. As you stop feeding an issue by not blocking yourself from it, it begins to slowly die, by processing its own negative energy. At this point, all you can do is put one foot in front of the other and get on with your day. Processing is not fun, but it is temporary and the way to permanently get rid of your dysfunction. If you think about it, when you've had an issue come up, you always felt it. It was an illusion that you could shield yourself from feeling it.

When negative compartments dissolve through The Practice, there simply is nothing to fend off. The ultimate form of inward protection is an awareness of what you see and knowing how to not protect yourself from yourself. In actuality, how can you protect yourself from yourself and who is the other self? The other self can only be a compartment and that's not you.

When your heart won't feel,
your pain can't heal.

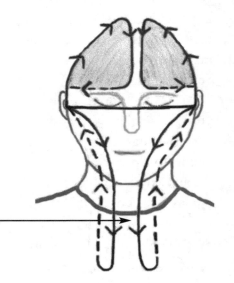

Emotional pain in your
heart pushes relationships
into your head

In relationships, you will only feel as close to another person as they are to their own heart. If a person has been deeply hurt or abused, an inability to relate with one's own heart will result in not allowing anyone close. If someone can't face his or her emotional hurt within, how can another get close?

If your heart is blocked by hurt, no one gets through the pain, and your relationships will move into your head. When you convince people you love them from your head, they won't feel love. When your head needs attention to feel wanted, you become high maintenance. No one outside you can ever give enough to make up for what you are absent of within—your connection to your heart.

The deepest hurt in your life will always reside in your greater Kelee with your conscious awareness being the recipient of the hurtful compartment. Your conscious awareness will try to protect itself, but if you cannot dissolve the compartment making your conscious awareness protective, you will not be open in your relationships. Your openness to life will suffer. This can only last so long, for anything that is not growing will stagnate and start dying.

Remember, when it comes to love, you can't have what you won't accept. The only recourse is to still your mind in your greater Kelee, so you can drop your mental protection and your pain can begin to heal.

Emotional pain is only an illusion that you are not worthy to be loved. How do you know you're worthy? If you have a heart, you most assuredly are!

*Attachment to love
is actually
the absence of love.*

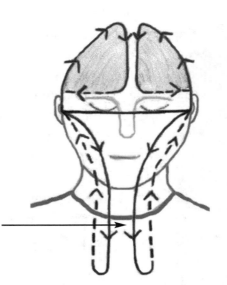

When compartments form in
the greater Kelee, you have
taken something to heart

The most painful experiences in life are the ones having to do with the giving and receiving of love. As human beings, we can endure a lot of pain as headaches, but when it comes to heartaches, a deep heartache can take down even the strongest of humans.

Everyone on the planet has probably heard the phrase, "You've taken something to heart." This is when you have taken into your greater Kelee another's negative perception of you and believed it. Someone else's negative view of you has become yours as a compartment.

Whenever you love someone and "keep them in your heart," you make a mental attachment to them. When mental attachments form, they compartmentalize. When the attachment is broken you feel broken. This is the proverbial heartache.

When love hurts, it's because you're holding onto something that was not yours to begin with. No one owns another's love. If you cannot detach from these compartmentalized attachments, they are excruciatingly painful. The Practice will dissolve these painful compartments, but why did you take them in to begin with? This is the deeper spiritual lesson having to do with the missing puzzle pieces in your spirit.

Heartaches end when self-acceptance starts. As you spend time in your heart through The Practice, you will understand why you hurt.

Remember, *love never hurts, the absence of love does.*

The map to understanding your heart is here, wouldn't it be wise to explore it?

To blindly trust
is an invitation to trouble.

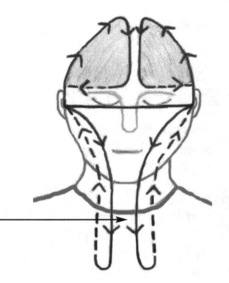

Trust is a perception your
spirit knows as accurate

The ultimate form of protection in life is learned by trusting what your conscious awareness senses. If you are to understand what you sense about others, you must understand yourself first. When you know how to open your spiritual senses, your newfound awareness will ultimately become your spiritual sight. When you learn how to read energy, you will understand that all energy is predictable.

If you meet someone for the first time and get a bad feeling, it's a warning. Beware, forewarned is forearmed. To give away trust is the mark of a fool, you will eventually be blind-sided.

Negativity always has a bad vibe and is very predictable. It causes trouble. Stay away from it. If you sense a negative compartment in someone and the compartment is stronger than that person's conscious awareness, trouble will come about. In fact, how do you trust people whose compartments are bigger than they are? You may be having a friendship with a compartment and not their spirit. You cannot trust compartments; they're mindless. If your friends are doing disharmonious things, maybe you need new friends. There is only so much time any of us can spend with others. Choose your friends wisely.

The Practice will open your eyes to many wonders but to be able to see them, you must learn to trust what you sense. As your mind becomes sharper over time through The Practice, you will begin to see and you'll be fascinated. As you begin to trust what you feel from your spirit, your ability to see will open from the darkness of unknowing, to the light of awareness. Trust your spirit, it can see beyond belief.

Wisdom
is determined by awareness,
not by age.

Age is determined by linear
thinking from the brain

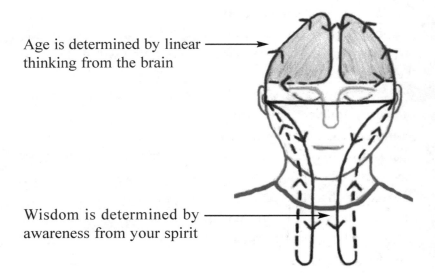

Wisdom is determined by
awareness from your spirit

Because you're old does not mean you'll be wise. So why is one person born with more wisdom than another? Why are kids who are raised by the same parents, in the same way, so different? Do parents determine a child's wisdom? This can't be true because some children grow up wiser than their parents.

Wisdom occurs because everyone's spirit is at a different level of awareness. This has nothing to do with fast firing neurons; intelligence has nothing to do with wisdom. Just because you have knowledge does not mean you'll know what to do with it. Wisdom is learned through experience and observation of what works and what does not.

Have you ever heard the expression, "He or she is an old soul." If there are old souls, then there must be young souls. How can this be? Whether you want to believe life is a one shot deal or you will live again, does not really matter. As your body ages, one day you will die. Then you'll realize that your spirit is non-physical and cannot die. What do you think happens to you when you die and what will you do? You will have to face this inevitable truth one day and I assure you, the adventure will continue! Wouldn't it be wise to explore your spirit now? Go inside your greater Kelee and you'll learn how.

Wisdom is the understanding of how to live harmoniously. Remember, this is your life we're talking about. Wise or foolish, it's your life to live.

Universal energy
is the energy of your spirit.

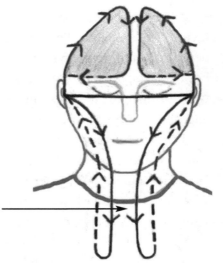

The energy of your spirit is
universal and unending

Universal energy is an endless supply of energy within your spirit. This energy can be felt most easily in your greater Kelee. The universal energy of your spirit is what brings you the feeling of connectedness and oneness with all things.

As you do The Practice, you'll begin to feel the sustaining universal energy of your spirit. Universal energy supports brain function, and runs mind function but does not feed dysfunction. When your conscious awareness is connected to your spirit, the physical energy of brain function can actually be tired without affecting mind function—which means you don't mentally crash. This is an extreme advantage when you have to be sharp, mentally strong and need endurance. Universal energy is the reason our spirit can't die. It's non-physical. We all have access to this stable form of unending energy if we know how to find it.

Do The Practice and over time you will feel this magnificent energy force. It will set your mind free and allow you to open to a new way of life you can't even imagine right now. If you want to master your mind i.e., spirit, you must learn to access this energy. The Kelee is a key to unlocking universal energy; all you need to do is allow your conscious awareness to feel it.

Look at how the energy of the Kelee folds in upon itself. The Kelee is like the universe itself, folding in upon itself without beginning or end. Universal energy flows through everything with awe-inspiring interaction. When it flows through you, you'll feel its presence, too!

When big sky mind is present,
you are!

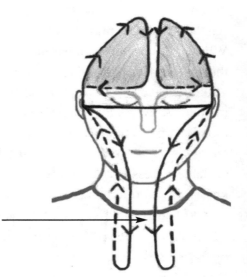

Big sky mind appears in
your greater Kelee as an
open blue sky

After doing The Practice diligently for some time, and when the time is right, you will attain a state of mind known as "big sky mind." It is a term used when your conscious awareness is in your greater Kelee and you feel free within your own mind. It is called big sky mind because when you're in this state of mind it feels like you're under the most magnificent blue sky you have ever seen. This incredible feeling of freedom occurs when you're not being bothered by interfering small mind chatter and from the absence of irritating compartments.

In this state of mind, you begin the realization process that is uninterrupted by negative thought. You begin to feel who you really are and realize that being open to the experience of life is a miracle.

You really can stand still and enjoy your own space. The space of your spirit opens you to a state of mindfulness that invites an exquisite way of being. There is no need to hurry from a place within you that feels better than any place outside you.

If you don't welcome yourself in your own mind, you won't feel welcome anywhere. The most beautiful part of big sky mind is once you find it, you take it everywhere you go. But alas, you will not attain big sky mind from the intellect by reading about it, but by being quiescent within your own mind.

There are many wonders in the world to explore and this state of mind will help you to explore them all with a light heart and a clear mind.

*When you see
the beauty of nature,
are you seeing its beauty
or your own?*

Chapter Seven

Your True Nature

When your true nature is open
to its significance
every moment of life
will have magnificence.

You cannot be someone
other than
who you really are.

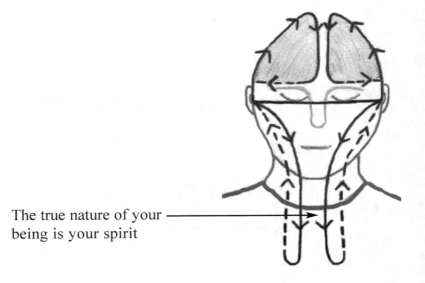

The true nature of your ────────── being is your spirit

The True Nature of Your Being

The true nature of your being is more about what it isn't, than what it is, because your spirit is non-physical and cannot be seen with your eyes. Do you ever wonder who you really are?

What you initially see in life comes from using your physical eyes, but the reality of how you live comes from your spirit. What you see is determined by how you perceive from your mind i.e., spirit, via the brain. It is said that the eyes are the windows to the soul but remember your eyes are only the windows, with your mind i.e., spirit, looking through them.

To find your spirit, you must learn how to sense it. You can sense with your five physical senses or your five spiritual ones. We each have a spiritual equivalent for each of the five physical senses. If you're only using your physical senses, you're only using half of your abilities. Can you imagine how much better your life would be if everything was twice as good as it is now, and that's just the start?

Many people have difficulty in understanding their mind i.e., spirit, because it's subtle in nature. If you are to develop your spirit, you must learn how to consciously open to it. As you do The Practice, you will find your true nature i.e., spirit, and believe it or not, it is within you, and there to be found in the Kelee.

Your spirit can open you to a life that is beyond imagination and yet it is truly the "real" of reality. If you want to get real, open to the true nature of you—your spirit.

You will not be happy
in the world
until you are happy
in yourself.

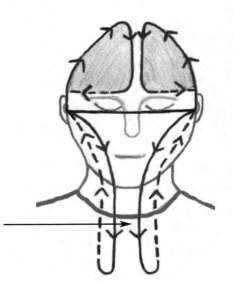

Happiness happens when
you feel alive in your spirit

If you're happy with yourself, you'll be happy anywhere. If you're not happy, why not? Maybe you're looking outside yourself to find happiness and are negating why you feel unhappy inside yourself?

When you experience happiness, you feel it. If you can't feel happiness, it means you're blocked from feeling it. The block to feeling happiness is compartments. Compartments are unhappy because they're not the real you. If you're not really you and you're not really living your life, how can you be happy with yourself?

Happiness is the absence of discontented compartments. Discontentment happens when a mindless compartment has decided how you feel. As compartments dissolve through The Practice, happiness appears in its place. The absence of dysfunction is always a reason for happiness.

If you look at when you're happy, it's always when you feel free in your mind. The minute you try to control happiness is the minute you stop experiencing it. Happiness is always when you feel like you're growing and learning. It's a warm feeling in your heart, open to the acceptance of a beautiful life. This warm place is a feeling of being alive and happens from being in your true nature.

Happiness is much more simple than people realize. Have you ever heard the expression, someone has a "happy heart." This is a clue to where happiness is found and guess where you need to look?

Contentment
is your mind's acceptance
of what life has to offer as beautiful.

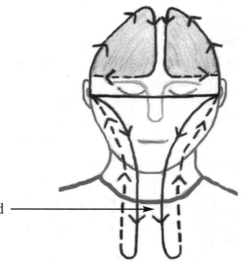

When life is not forced
contentment happens
naturally

Contentment happens when your mind is free from need and you're feeling carefree. You experience the world with the awe of a child. Your spiritual eyes are open and the world looks like a garden. Everything around you gently interacts as the wind blows through the trees, butterflies float by and clouds drift along under a blue sky. There's no separation between your true nature and the physical world around you.

True contentment is the need for nothing outside you. When your true nature sustains you, contentment fulfills need and want. What you have been seeking has always been within you. *Contentment happens when you accept your mind as beautiful.*

How you find contentment is by living your experience of life through your own mind. When your mind is open to life and you're not distracted by the brain, and not disturbed by compartments, contentment will follow.

When your spirit is fulfilled and your cup is overflowing with contentment, what more can be given to you?

If you could buy contentment, how much would it be worth to you?

Being contented feels like someone is paying you to live your life in paradise. It is a beautiful way of being. Simply put, contentment is you liking yourself.

The most successful moments of life
are always
the ones you enjoyed.

Success in the intellect is
security and materialization

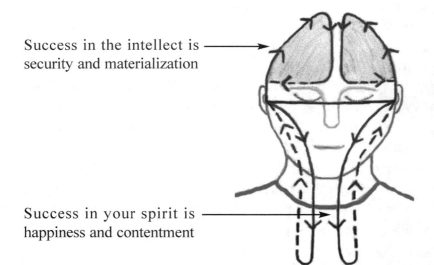

Success in your spirit is
happiness and contentment

Success is experienced in two basic forms: material and spiritual. The dysfunction from compartments always gets in the way of both forms of success; they interfere with your work and they interfere with your home. Compartments do not discriminate what area of your life they steal energy from; they will suck the life right out of you. When your life sucks, compartments are the culprit!

The Practice will eventually dissolve the problem of compartments, but you still must learn how to delegate your time. Whenever you put too much time into the outside world, your inside world suffers and the spiritual law of balance i.e., moderation, is broken. Balancing your time between work and home is extremely important. You must have time to yourself at home to be successful at work. Time away from work is just as important as time at work. If your home is a wreck, it's only a matter of time before your work will be too.

Home is where your heart is. If your heart is not in what you do, does what you do even matter? If you don't feel your own success, who will?

Success is not complete until you feel it.

When your heart is happy, being unsuccessful doesn't even enter your mind. The bottom line with success is this, if you're enjoying what you do, you do it well.

When the mind is empty to receive,
acceptance of life
becomes fulfillment.

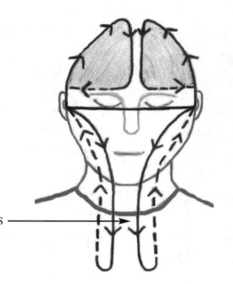

Emptiness of compartments
is openness to fulfillment
from your spirit

The Emptiness of Fulfillment

When your greater and lesser Kelee are not crowded with compartments consuming you with negativity, spiritual emptiness happens. This feeling of emptiness gives you space to breathe and in itself is incredible, giving you a feeling of freedom and allowing you to be who you really are. As you begin to settle down and enjoy this freedom, an amazing thing happens. You realize the space within you is not just empty space, but has a beautiful feeling of contentment to it. It is your true nature—your spirit—and feels better than anything the intellect can imagine. Your spirit naturally feels good because it does not have the constriction of mass.

As you do The Practice, your heart starts to open up and it feels much better than living in your head. When you hear the term "being open," this is it. The being nature of your spirit is open to accepting the experience of life. This is when each moment feels new as it passes through your spirit. This is "the now" everyone is trying to find, but it's not accessed from the intellect, it's experienced by opening to the empty space of your spirit.

This beautiful form of spiritual emptiness is the openness to fulfillment. It is complete acceptance of experience and it feels harmonious. Harmony is opening up, negativity is closing down.

Harmony always offers more knowledge of life than negativity.

When you allow life to flow, it will flow through you. You feel alive, fulfilled, and everything feels in its place. How would you like to live in this space? Do The Practice and you will.

*When you're vulnerable to hurt
you close down.
When you're vulnerable to love
you open up.*

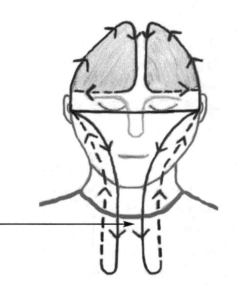

When you're vulnerable
to love, you open to love

Vulnerability is associated with feeling a need to protect yourself in two ways: from physical harm or emotional pain. Physical harm is relatively easy to deal with by removing yourself from the potential danger. However, when it comes to protecting yourself from emotional pain, it's completely different. How do you do that? How do you protect yourself from something you can't see and only feel?

There are two types of emotional pain: yours and another's. The only way to protect yourself from your own emotional pain is with awareness. This is learned through detachment, by living within your own mind i.e., spirit, at all times.

The Practice will teach you how to deal with your own pain but when it comes to another's emotional pain, you'll need to pay attention. The moment you become aware that you're feeling another's emotional pain is the moment you are most vulnerable to accepting it as yours. You must learn how to protect yourself from the emotional pain of others without blocking your experience of life. You do this by allowing another their own space. If someone's emotional instability is simply too painful to be around, don't be there. The people in our life are a choice. Harmonious people promote happiness, and disharmonious people promote suffering.

When your conscious awareness feels vulnerable, it's called being open to yourself. It will take bravery to face whether or not you feel worthy to be loved. If you love who you are, who can stop you from feeling it?

When you're vulnerable to love, the paradise of your true nature awaits.

The heart of your being
is your spirit.
Who would have guessed?

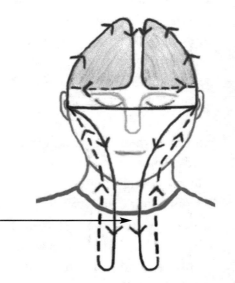

The heart of your being is
your conscious awareness
centered here

When we talk about love and our heart, we're not talking about our physical heart, we're referring to the heart of our being—our spirit. When we're in our heart it is recognized by all to be a good thing. However, have you noticed that your heart can feel emotional pain or it can feel love?

If love never hurts, why does your heart hurt sometimes? Your heart hurts because it's open to the pain of compartments.

If you want to feel love in your heart, you must be open to your mind i.e., spirit. If you look at what your heart really is, it is your conscious awareness being open to your spirit. Remember, your mind i.e., spirit, has conscious awareness; your brain i.e., intellect, has sense-consciousness. Compartments have no consciousness.

The heart of your being is centered in your greater Kelee. That's why, when you feel love, you feel it in this place. Look at the Kelee drawing. You've felt emotion in this place. Everyone has! As you begin to do The Practice, your heart will become more familiar to you. After all it is you.

There are many questions to answer on your spiritual path, but the deepest and most profound realizations are about your heart and your relationship with love. The way to find your answers to love is by being in your greater Kelee with your conscious awareness open and receptive. From stilling your conscious awareness in your greater Kelee, clarity from stillness will bring forth your answers.

When your heart is open to love, love opens you to life.

If you want love in your life, open your conscious awareness to the heart of your being, otherwise known as the greater Kelee.

Love
is the beautiful self-acceptance
of who we really are.

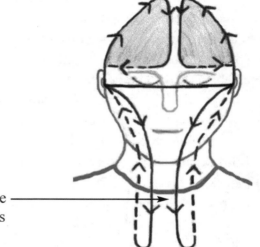

Love never hurts, the
absence of love does

People love in two ways, with only one way being real. One way is from your head and the other is from your heart. Guess which one is real.

When people love from their head, it always feels cold. It's much more like a business deal. If you do this for me, I'll do that for you. This supposed way of love always has expectations, which is the prelude to emotional hurt and pain.

When you try to love from your head, it's because you're not feeling it from your heart. Your head may try to give love but it ends up projecting expectations of what you need. The need to mentally control how another loves you is possessiveness. Possessiveness forms attachments, which when broken makes you feel broken and is extremely painful.

What you need from others is what you really need to feel in yourself—love.

If you want to love another but don't love yourself, what can you give?

The greatest gift you can give to another is sharing your own loving presence. What you bring to a relationship is what's in your heart and when it's love, the absence of separation is felt and your relationship feels beautiful. There is an old saying, "Two minds can never be as one, but they can touch softly."

Everyone wants to feel love, but the acceptance of it must start with you. Remember, love is born when you realize your true nature is beautiful. Your self-acceptance of this beauty is what warms your heart and opens you to love.

*The beauty of a loving touch
is heaven on earth.*

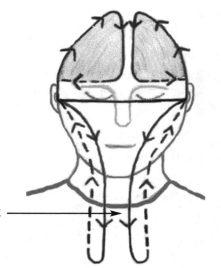

A loving touch is the highest
expression of life from the
physical

Sexuality in a healthy state of mind can be one of the most beautiful experiences we can have with someone we love. When we are touched with a hand that is warm with love, it's a heavenly experience. When your hand touches another from your heart, it is the highest physical expression you can have.

Sexuality when experienced from your heart is a beautiful part of nature and from a purely physiological standpoint, is necessary for your health. If you do not have periodical releases, you can develop any number of diseases in your reproductive organs. When energy is not passing through all parts of the body at a moderate rate, stagnation occurs and disease right behind that. When your mind and body are moving into harmony, disharmony is dispelled.

When your true nature regulates your brain and compartments, life is easier, less complicated and more beautiful. Invariably problems with sexuality will manifest as compartments because of missing spiritual puzzle pieces. Imprint this in your intellect: if you're not comfortable with your sexuality, know that you are not flawed, only experiencing an unrealized part of your spirit. All sexual problems blocking your ability to feel good about yourself will eventually be solved by your spirit.

When each person cleans up their own mind, so-called dirty thoughts do not occur. The beauty of a loving touch is our birthright. If you do not enjoy your sexuality, isn't it time to start?

There's nothing ugly about sexuality, except your own misperception of what physical beauty really is.

*Peace on earth
will only happen
when we as people are peaceful within.*

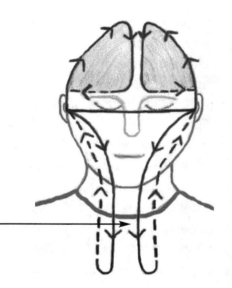

Peace is an uninterrupted
space within your own
mind i.e., spirit

Human beings are the most advanced life form on the planet. Or are we? If each individual in the world does not know how to find a peaceful state of mind, we will collectively never have a peaceful place to live. A peaceful life isn't found outside you, it's experienced within you.

If a person cannot feel their spirit, they invariably will create an ego to replace it. Ego is an artificial you, which has a need to control because it feels inferior, disconnected and destitute. No one's spirit is inferior or superior; we're all simply learning who we are as humans.

When you come to terms with yourself, you'll begin to find the answers to your own questions. The world does not hold your answers, your own mind does. Problems in the mind always comes from the place it starts—compartments. Compartments are ultimately the reason for disharmony. They're mindless. They make no sense at all and yet people live by them.

As the space within your Kelee becomes increasingly open, you will feel the uninterrupted space of peace in your spirit. When you live peacefully, you will help others without even trying, by example of your peaceful nature. There is a phrase from my first book, *The Way is Within,* that says it all: "Be at peace with yourself, if you are not at peace with yourself, you are at peace with nothing."

If mankind does not follow the spiritual law of harmony i.e., non-interference, suffering will continue on the planet. End your suffering and you will not contribute to the world's.

When you are no better than dirt,
you will honor walking on it.

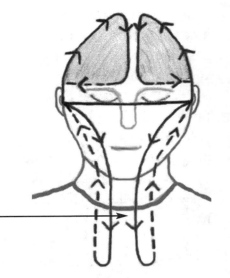

Humbleness is grateful
appreciation in your spirit

To value the best in life, you must have an appreciation for the least. To understand humbleness, you must learn why it is important to sweep the steps to your own house. When you are no better than the dirt you sweep, you are worthy to walk on it. We are born of the earth, live from the earth and will go back to it one day. Humbleness is the grateful acceptance of simplistic beauty.

Most of your life is spent doing mundane things; it would be wise to enjoy them. When you're living from your true nature, you do not need outside recognition. All of what you do has significance one way or another if you're aware. If you're not aware of how you're living, does what you do even matter?

Take the time to observe the simplicity of nature and how it interacts harmoniously. Everything in nature has a purpose. Pay attention to the simple beauty in nature and you will begin to feel your place in it. You will begin to sense contentment, which is a feeling that, "I belong here."

We are all a part of this same nature, if we can feel it. I know a master who can do anything you can imagine, and he loves to watch ants. The root of spirituality is an understanding that everything is relevant. If you don't care, you don't feel. If you don't feel, you don't love. What's the point of living without a loving experience of life?

You only appreciate the highest life has to offer by understanding the steps of the lowest first.

*The magic kingdom
is only as real
as your ability to experience its beauty.*

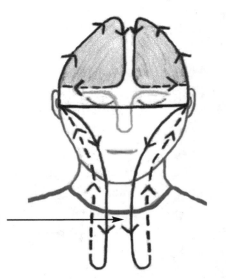

The magic kingdom appears
when your spirit sees the
world

When you have done The Practice for a while and the time is right, a magical event occurs—your spiritual eyes open to the world.

When you have taken off the blinders of belief, the magic kingdom miraculously appears before you. You become light on your feet, have joy in your heart, your eyes have the wonder of a child and everything looks new. The sky is bluer, trees are greener, flowers appear brighter, and it's as if, with a clear pen, someone has outlined everything in life with clarity. You become a living breathing interacting participant in life. You feel life with every fiber of your being; there is no separation between you and the world around you. You feel as if you're on some magical drug, but it's completely natural. When this happens, it's like walking into a magic kingdom. It's a place where you feel free in your mind and the world is an exquisitely beautiful place to be. This place is the proverbial "Kingdom of God." It's not a way to believe, it's a way to live from your spirit here and now. It's a kingdom within your mind that brings life alive.

Truly, the world is determined by your mind. You are not determined by the world. The world outside does not see through your eyes; you perceive the world from your spiritual eyes. If the spiritual world is invisible to you, it's because you're seeing through your physical eyes, not your spiritual ones.

If you do The Practice, one day your spiritual eyes will open and you'll enter a state of mind where you feel forever young and everything is always beautiful.

*Spiritual truth
is a gentle breeze,
not a howling wind.*

Chapter Eight
Spiritual Truths

There is nothing
that can defile your spirit
only the appearance
that it can.

*Change
is the spiritual law
of impermanence.*

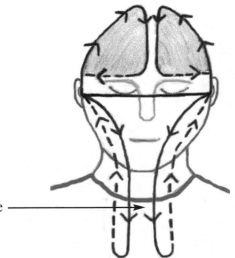

The mind accepts change
when it does not fear it

There is an old saying, "Change is the only constant in the universe." When you're afraid to change, it's because you fear what you're changing into will be worse than how you are now. While this can be true if you're unaware, it does not have to be.

If you're filled with compartments, change is difficult because compartments are self-sustaining, fearful time capsules. Each time you try to replicate an experience, something is lost until these created comfort zones become a control issue. Controlling change is an illusion. Ironically, *the more you try to hold things together, the easier they fall apart.*

As your compartments begin to disappear through The Practice, fear is dissolved, allowing you to embrace transitions without worrying about whether the experience will measure up to your expectations. If you want to get rid of worry, get rid of compartments. They fear newness.

As you begin to open to your mind i.e., spirit, in your greater Kelee, freedom from fear starts happening because your spirit accepts change and it welcomes new experiences, which means growth. If you fight change, you will find yourself in a battle of frustration.

You cannot hold back change; anything that is not growing is in a process of dying. Life depends on change. All masters understand that wisdom is the acceptance of change.

There is only one good way to deal with change, enjoy it.

*No distractions
is the spiritual law
of mindfulness.*

The biggest distractions in
the world are the ones in
your own mind

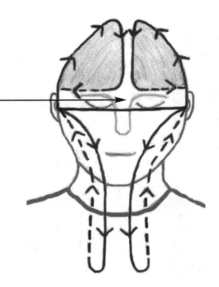

You can walk away from the distractions outside you, but you cannot walk away from the ones within you. If you are distracted, how can you do what you want to do?

The three big distractions are:

1. **Distractions from sense-consciousness in the brain:** avoiding pain and seeking pleasure with your physical senses to excess.

2. **Distractions from the world of people, places and things:** spending excessive amounts of time on things other than your own mind.

3. **Distractions from compartments in your Kelee:** when compartments within your own mind control your life.

The spiritual law of moderation will take care of sense-consciousness distractions. However, the most bothersome distractions will come from within you as compartments that have a mind of their own. Your mind may have one thought on what to do and a compartment has another. Which one wins out? If the compartment is stronger than your conscious awareness, you will not end up doing what you want to do. If you're not doing what you want to do, who's in control? This is actually easy to solve through The Practice. When the compartment dissolves, you're in control.

As you do The Practice, your mind will find freedom from distractions, this is the nature of your spirit. When you're not distracted, you're mindful.

*Moderation
is the spiritual law
of balance.*

Moderation is the balance
point of your soul

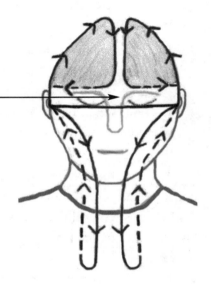

There are two basic forms of balance: physical and spiritual. If you eat too much, drink too much, work too much, you suffer. Anything that becomes excessive having to do with sense-consciousness and your physical shell will turn from abundance to suffering. Mankind's brain seems to have a curse on it, because it can never get enough and yet it can only have half.

When you learn how to live from your spirit more than your brain, you will start to understand sense-consciousness cravings. Deeper than the cravings are why they control you—a missing spiritual puzzle piece. Substance abuse is one of the puzzle pieces that everyone will have to master, or suffering will continue relentlessly until you do.

Remember, controlling substance abuse is more about controlling you, rather than the substance. A substance cannot jump into your mouth by itself. You put it in there and if it's hurting you, you need to know why. If you want to be balanced in the physical, moderation is the way to be in harmony with your body.

If your body feels balanced but your spirit does not, it's because your conscious awareness is leaning too far forward into the future or leaning too far back into your past. It is always when you're not paying attention to the moment, that you lose your balance and fall.

Moderation is one of the important keys to harmony; it would be wise to be mindful of this spiritual law. Follow it and you're blessed, ignore it and you feel cursed.

*Non-interference
is the spiritual law
of harmony!*

Non-interference is the way
of harmony in the mind

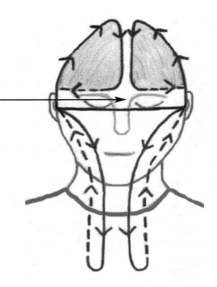

Non-interference is the most important spiritual law in the universe. Interference is when you deliberately try to control another's life. It is simply wrong to do this in any way, shape or form! If no one ever broke this spiritual law, there would be no disharmony between individuals.

People interfere in two basic ways: intentionally by deliberately interfering and unintentionally through ignorance from unknowing. Whether you interfere intentionally or unintentionally, you set into motion another spiritual law—karma or cause and effect.

When you don't set negativity into motion, you won't have to deal with it. If you're not interfering with others, you can focus on living your own life. When you learn to live your own life, you will begin to understand it. Everyone has a path to walk, and it is up to each one of us to decide what we are here to do.

As you do The Practice, you will find yourself living more within your own mind. You will realize that it doesn't feel good to put your clean hand into something that is not. Why would you want to be touching someone else's negativity, otherwise known as compartments? Are you trying to fix them, and how exactly are you going to do that? Whom have you ever fixed? It would be more important to ask yourself why you need to solve another's problems.

It's amazing, when you leave people alone, they like it. This is the understanding of the spiritual law of harmony—non-interference.

Karma
is the spiritual law
of cause and effect.

What your conscious
awareness sows, it reaps

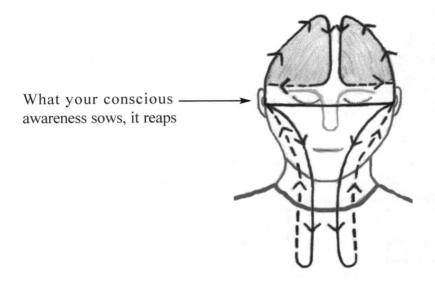

It is said that a butterfly can flap its wings on one side of the world and change the weather on the other side. For every action, there will be a reaction somewhere. While this is a metaphor for how interconnected everything is, there is a grain of truth in it. Nature is going to do what it's going to do, according to natural law. Fighting with nature is futile. The only recourse is to understand and flow with it.

Understanding karma comes from understanding your conscious awareness and the true nature of your own mind. What is your conscious awareness doing at any given moment? This moment is where you set karma in motion, harmonious or disharmonious.

If you pay attention, you'll notice karma also involves the spiritual law of mindfulness—no distractions. If you're distracted, you may set something in motion that you don't want to happen. This can involve others. This can affect the spiritual law of harmony—non-interference. If you're not in harmony, this involves the spiritual law of love and that of abundance. If you break spiritual law it is easy to see how downward spirals are caused and affect you.

Your mind is responsible for everything you think and feel. This is why awareness is so important. If a thought compartmentalizes as disharmony, you will be forced to deal with it as your karma one way or another; this is an absolute. *You get away with nothing in the mind.*

What your mind sows, it reaps. Remember, bad karma is only a lack of mindfulness, not a curse. Bad karma ends when you stop causing it.

*Kindness
is the warmth
that allows us to care.*

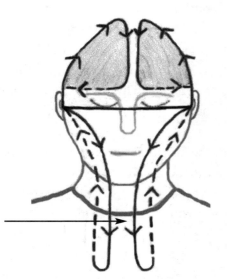

Kindness in your heart will
heal any wound imaginable
in your soul

To be kind to anyone, you must first be kind to yourself. When you don't care for yourself, you will not care about anything. What kind of life is that? It seems that for most people it is easier to beat yourself up than to be kind to yourself. Does this make any sense?

Once at a difficult time in my life, when I was hurting and as down as I could get, I went to see a wise teacher. He looked at me and with his gentle, caring eyes said an extremely profound statement that I will never forget, *"Oh my son, what are you doing? Be kind to yourself."* Anytime when I am troubled, I think about his words, which still bring tears of gratitude to my eyes. I was so thankful that someone would treat me with such kindness and care.

The kindest thing you can do for yourself is to do The Practice. Each time you sit down and still your mind, you care for your mind. This care one day will be the care you can share with others.

Be kind to yourself. Imprint this on your brain, so as not to forget when you can't reach your heart in time of need.

When you forgive yourself, you will be forgiven and the suffering ends. There is absolutely nothing which you regret, that your heart can't heal. Go into your heart and feel kindness for yourself and your life will change forever.

If you do not condemn people,
you will never need to forgive them.

If you're holding contempt ———→
for another, it's your problem
not theirs

Whenever you do something to hurt another human being, at the deepest point in your spirit, you don't really want to do it. It feels wrong. Whenever someone intentionally hurts you, it is their karma—cause and effect—to deal with, not yours. When you have this understanding, it will set you free.

The trail of hurt always leads back to the one inflicting it. If you condemn someone who inflicts their pain on you, who is walking around with the condemnation? Have you ever had the thought that you could be walking around with a compartment, condemning someone and the person you're condemning doesn't even know it? Who's stuck with what? Sadly enough, even if you try to forgive someone from your head, you still feel hurt. You won't feel free.

Making mistakes is often a part of learning. You have probably done more stupid things than you can count. Who hasn't? Whenever you do something wrong, on some level you always know it. It feels wrong!

If you're not paying attention to how you really feel, you're blocking your feelings. If you fear you're not worthy of being loved, you will not want to feel your own painful compartments. What you may not understand is that your emotional pain is not you. It would be wise to find out why you have it.

If you don't forgive yourself, you won't forgive others. Trust your feelings as being what they are and you will learn that emotional pain belongs to no one's spirit.

Like attracts like
is the spiritual law
of compatibility.

An ego and compartments
are compatible with no
one, including you

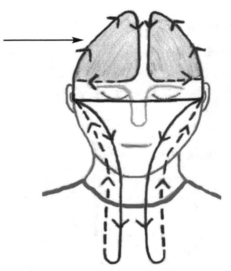

When it comes to people, not everyone is compatible in the same place at the same time. You will not be simpatico with everyone and there is not much you can do about it, except be someplace else. That's just the way it is until you understand what's causing the separation.

There are two main reasons people are incompatible: egos and compartments.

The reason people create an ego is because their conscious awareness cannot feel their spirit, so they create what they think life is and end up separating themselves from life, which causes disharmony. You cannot be compatible with people who are not compatible with themselves.

Compartments are another reason for incompatibility. As you do The Practice and clear yourself of compartments, you become aware of how many people are filled with them. If you are around someone who has great difficulty because of their compartments, they will bring their difficulty into your life.

The darkness of ignorance and the light of awareness do not share the same space. There will be a reaction, one way or another when these two forces meet. The darkness of ignorance is always unaware of the trouble it causes because it lives in it. Why subject yourself to this lesser way of being and for what reason? This is not a judgment; it's having the freedom to choose where you place yourself.

People are incompatible because they haven't dealt with their issues! You only have so much time, remember; friends are a choice, not an obligation. Choose wisely.

Love
is the spiritual law
of abundance.

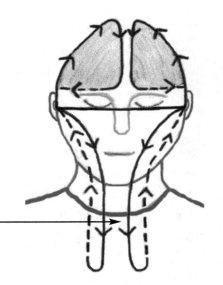

Love is not found in your
physical heart, it's found in
your spiritual one

The spiritual law of love is a law that we as humans cannot live without. Without a question, love is the most sought-after feeling on the planet. When you're truly in love, you want for nothing. This is the nature of the abundance of love.

You may have everything in the outside world, but it means nothing if your spirit feels devoid of love. It may seem strange that love is actually a spiritual law, but can you imagine living a life without it? Isn't the disharmony in the world because of a lack of love?

To have the abundance of love, your heart must be open. Where this openness is found is within your own spirit. The place to feel love has always been known. You know it yourself, you've felt it in your own heart. Look at the diagram. Isn't this the same place you have always felt love?

If you really look at what love is, it is your own beautiful self-acceptance of your own heart. If you cannot accept yourself, what can be given to you by another? If you can't feel your own heart, how can you feel another's love?

What if you want to love another but can't open your own heart? The Practice will open your heart, if you take the time to go inside and get still. The directions to your heart will never be so clear as what you see right now.

When you embrace the beautiful nature of your spirit, you will learn to accept love. When you accept love in your own heart, you can accept the love of others.

*Each one of us
is here to do something,
that's endearing to our soul.*

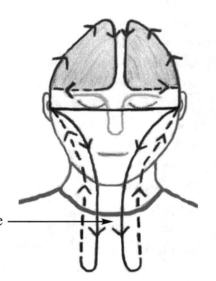

Your niche isn't found outside
you; it's realized inside you

The three big questions in life are: Who am I? Why am I here? And where am I going?

To find your niche, where do you look? The place to start your search is not out in the world, it's within your own mind. Truly to find your niche, you must find yourself first. However, you aren't found outside yourself, you find yourself inside yourself.

What are you here to do? And how can you find what you want to do if you don't know what you want to do? Discovering your likes is the first step to finding your niche. This is done by learning what touches your mind i.e., spirit. If you don't know your likes, explore until you do. Remember, *your niche is found by what feels good to you, not what feels good to other people.*

If you can't feel your niche right now, there is an old saying, "chop wood and carry water." In other words, do what you need to do in your day with your awareness wide open and when you're ready, a particular feeling will dawn upon you, and you will realize what your niche is.

A niche is a soulful blending of doing and being— when what you do is an extension from your being in a harmonious relationship with life. In actuality, you are your niche.

When you are truly happy with what you do, you will have found your niche.

*Don't worry
about where you're going,
pay attention to where you are.*

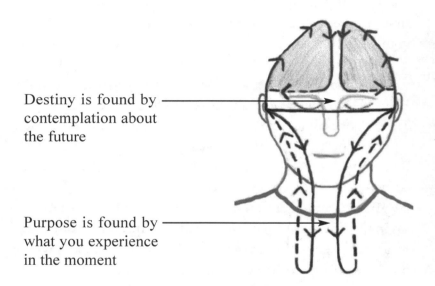

Destiny is found by
contemplation about
the future

Purpose is found by
what you experience
in the moment

When we think about our destiny, it always seems to be about what's to come, in the future. To most people, it seems as if there's a question as to who's in control of our destiny. Truly, your destiny is up to you. You must find your own way. Who can walk your feet for you? Remember, on your pathway through life, most of your attention should be on your next couple of steps and only occasionally on looking up to see if you're going the direction you want to go.

If you look within your own heart, you will feel your true nature and understand that we all have a purpose that eventually leads to our individual destinies. When you begin to understand you have a purpose, you will notice that you always *feel* it in the moment. This is the first step to your destiny.

Sometimes in your life, *you just know things* and when you pay attention and follow through, you begin to learn how you know things. This is awareness. When you begin to really live each moment, your purpose will become clear; when you have a purpose, you have a destiny ahead! Remember, *a purpose is fulfilled each time you enjoy doing something.*

The Practice has ended up being my destiny. But if you look at my work carefully, it is a collective of individual realizations over time that has brought about a purpose for living that has lead to my individual destiny.

Everyone is destined for greatness one day and yes, it is found in each purposeful step.

*In a single moment of time
self-realization can happen.
What allows it to happen
is acceptance of knowledge
without changing it.*

Chapter Nine

Spiritual Puzzle Pieces

*Inspiration is
your spirit's longing
to fulfill itself
in the deepest sense,
finding your
spiritual puzzle pieces.*

Self-realization
is the process of understanding
who you really are,
otherwise known as enlightenment.

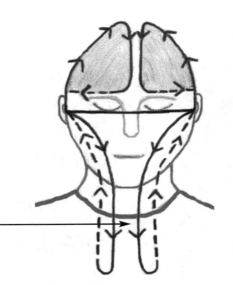

The realization of your
spirit is the understanding
of your spirit

The understanding of your spirit is a journey with a destiny of realizing completeness. The spiritual path is the journey that brings the opportunity to realize why you suffer—the result of having missing spiritual puzzle pieces.

In the bigger picture of enlightenment, a question often arises. "How many spiritual puzzle pieces do I need to be complete?" There is no set number because your own mind is determining how you perceive what you're missing. What one person might perceive as one big puzzle piece, another person might perceive as five smaller ones, so the number with each person is a variable.

We all must learn the same lessons to free ourselves, but how we perceive them is up to us individually. Each individual puzzle piece is as important as the complete picture because you cannot have one without the other. This is why the journey is everything. The joy of finding each puzzle piece is the adventure of life. If you are to find your missing spiritual puzzle pieces, you must be open to experience them directly from your spirit.

The Practice is a pathway that opens you to your heart and leads you to your spirit. This knowledge is as clear as the sunrise, but it is only you who can decide to open your eyes to see it.

What everyone is looking for comes by means of your mind i.e., spirit. Isn't it time to experience the pathway you came here to walk?

*The spiritual path
is not an intellectualization,
it's a search
for your missing spiritual puzzle pieces.*

Your intellect believes
because it does not know

Your spirit knows because
it does not have to believe

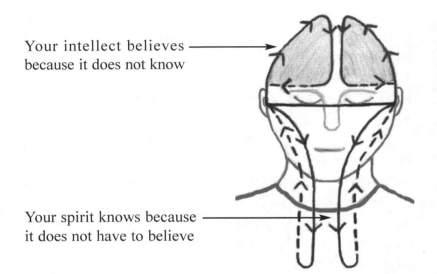

If you have not had the personal experience to understand knowing, you will be forced to believe something until you do. For example, you can read all you want about love, but until you have had the real experience, you know nothing.

Everyone must get out of his or her head and into their heart to love. When we talk about being in our head or our heart, it is a literal place found in the Kelee. I am sure we can all agree that being a loving being is at the heart of being spiritual, with the greater Kelee being where we feel love.

How do you translate conceptual knowledge into a loving experience of life? Can intellectual religion teach you to love? Truly, love precedes all religions. When it does not, then dogma has replaced love.

Through doing The Practice and by dissolving compartments, you will simply begin to dissolve the blocks to love. Then you will not have to override the blocks and try to believe in love, you can experience love directly for yourself. No one can love for you, you must feel it yourself.

What everyone is trying to find on a spiritual path is the missing pieces of their spiritual puzzle. If you just read this book without doing The Practice, you will never understand it. The spiritual path is actually quite simple: get out of the theories from your head, get rid of your blocks i.e., compartments, and open to your spirit. What you'll experience will amaze you!

Spiritual puzzle pieces
are the realization
of why we no longer need to suffer.

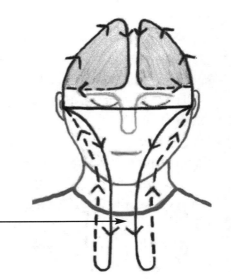

The realization of puzzle
pieces is the beginning of
the end of suffering

Spiritual puzzle pieces are difficult to describe because they're innate feelings of knowledge in your spirit. Trying to describe a feeling with words is like trying to describe love without feeling it.

Have you ever noticed that your head can think without feeling and your spirit can feel without thinking? One day, you must decide where you trust from, your head or your heart. Ponder this, *you think what you don't know, but feel what you do.* Whenever you think you know, you're always uncertain. Knowing always comes down to a feeling process, just like love.

The foundation of love is found in self-acceptance of your spirit. Self-acceptance is the place you will eventually end up when you stop trying to take from others what is rightfully yours, the ability to feel love in yourself. When you experience love for what it really is, you will realize that love can only come from your own self-acceptance of it.

Feeling your heart is the opening of self-acceptance. Why would you not accept yourself? You're here, aren't you? Why do people feel so unworthy and need validation from others? Why do people so desperately seek love from others? Can it be you don't feel love within?

The deeper reason for suffering is always missing puzzle pieces. What you're looking for is to complete yourself by understanding what's separating you from your openness to life.

When your own self-acceptance is in place, you will never feel misplaced again.

Theories don't complete us,
realizations
known as spiritual puzzle pieces do.

Your brain theorizes
because you have not
had direct experience

Your spirit realizes
because you have had
direct experience

The quandary everyone's trying to solve is how to free themselves from their internal difficulties and how to be a loving being. The reason you pick up a difficulty i.e., a compartment, is your spirit doesn't know not to because of a missing piece of your spiritual puzzle. If your conscious awareness does not understand something about yourself, you will either theorize what to do or follow what someone else has done.

True self-understanding cannot come from theory but by opening your mind—spirit—directly to life. Opening your mind can be scary because it means you must be responsible for yourself. Your head can theorize and justify away emotional pain, but if you do something wrong from your heart and know it, it can be devastating. If you're not brave enough to learn from your spirit, you will not grow and will forever run from that which imposes upon you. *Our spirit is not here to impose on us, but invites us to explore it.*

As you do The Practice and dissolve compartments blocking you from life, your spirit will open naturally without fear. When your spirit has an uninterrupted experience of life, you'll feel it directly. When your mind i.e., spirit, sees clearly, you will realize what not to do and a spiritual puzzle piece will be born.

The greatest puzzle in the universe to complete is your own. Want to play?

When you pick up baggage,
it's because you don't realize
that what you're picking up
is not yours.

Compartments are the
baggage of your soul

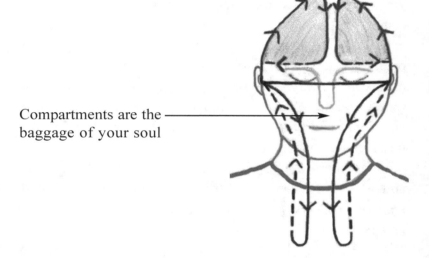

As you live your life, it's quite natural to touch things to investigate them. Everyone's spirit is curious by nature. If what your mind touches feels good and you can let go of it—there's no problem—but if what you touch is negative and your mind can't let go, it becomes yours in your Kelee.

Taking on baggage is a real Catch-22 situation. If you don't know how not to pick up something negative, how do you stop yourself? If your compartments are blocking you from what you need to learn, how do you get rid of the blocks to learn? The Practice will solve this problem, not to worry.

Think of picking up baggage as a pointer to something you are here to learn about. You picked up the baggage because you have missing spiritual puzzle pieces associated with that baggage. If you have an issue with something, you have a missing puzzle piece deeper in your spirit. These unrealized parts of your spirit are the solution to all of the problems you have created for yourself. Finding these spiritual lessons is a process of spiritual growth that brings you alive.

Wouldn't it be great if you felt like you were always on vacation? Why can't you enjoy life all of the time? When baggage is dropped through The Practice, your conscious awareness will operate without blocks in the way. Then it can feel like you're on a vacation every day.

When you realize from your spirit why you picked up baggage, you will never pick up that particular compartment ever again!

*A commitment
is only as valuable
as your ability to keep it.*

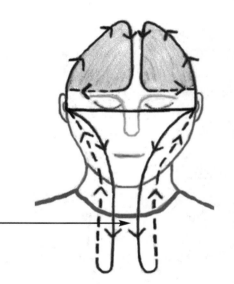

The greatest commitment
you will ever make is to
know yourself

When you make a commitment to help yourself from your head and fail, it's because your heart wasn't into it. You may have had good intentions from your head, but lack the patience and follow-through that your spirit can provide.

Commitments work when your word is grounded in your heart i.e., spirit, not in compartments. *Your word is everything.* If your word isn't sound, how sound are you?

The greatest commitment you will ever make will be to know yourself. If you don't know yourself, can you be trusted? This is not easy to look at, but if you don't know and trust your own spirit, you will forever struggle with issues relating to reliability and truthfulness.

Mistrust in yourself is really misperception influenced by compartments that produce failed commitments. If a fearful compartment is where a commitment came from, you can be sure you'll struggle with the process of keeping your word.

Remember, it's your conscious awareness that determines what commitments come out of your mouth, trustworthy or not! It would be wise to know your thoughts before you make any promises. A quiet mind is the foundation for clarity of thought; all good commitments start from this place.

Self-commitment is a state of mind that it would be wise to find sooner rather than later. Commit to doing The Practice and you will learn why your commitments are, or are not, always beautiful and truthful.

When you're in denial
of your own problems,
they become everyone else's.

Denial is a refusal to see ⟶
your own compartments

If you're not responsible for your actions, they become someone else's problem to deal with. Self-denial is a refusal to see what you cannot escape—yourself.

When your conscious awareness does not want to face an issue, i.e., a compartment, you will normally throw up a wall to protect yourself from feeling a compartment that you have mistaken as you. Protecting yourself from what you have mistakenly believed is you is a lack of awareness. If you cannot be yourself because a compartment is threatening your conscious awareness, you will have to escape somehow. No one can ever block out a compartment for long; the compartment will rear its ugly head. Compartments always do. They are not to be trusted!

If someone around you is in denial and you call them on it, they most often will turn the situation around and make you feel as if you've done something wrong or it's your problem. If you force the issue, you may hear the phrase, "I'm not going there." This is where the conversation will end if the wall of denial is too strong. Don't push it. Resistance is futile at this point.

The only way out of denial is with the light of awareness through the realization that we have nothing to be ashamed of in our spirit. Each time you still your mind, you drop the walls protecting your issues. When your issues get weaker, your conscious awareness grows stronger.

If someone around you points out your denial, don't close the door—open it. You might learn something. It could be the puzzle piece you need to stop self-denial once and for all.

*Addiction is a craving to find
what only
your spirit can fulfill.*

Addiction is the brain living
without fulfillment from your
spirit

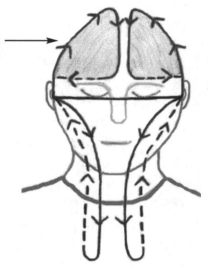

If you have an addictive personality, your brain operates without direction from your mind i.e, spirit—you have a missing spiritual puzzle piece. If you don't know how to experience from your spirit, you will be subject to the brain's need to avoid emotional pain and seek sense consciousness pleasures to excess. This breaks the spiritual law of balance —moderation, and suffering begins.

Addiction is all about getting a physical feeling. The problem starts when you feel through the body only; there's never enough and it does not last. If you can't feel life with your spirit, then you will substitute with something else.

When you can move out of sense consciousness from the brain and into the space of your spirit, fulfillment can begin to end the suffering from addiction. Ending substance abuse is about understanding why you would allow something that has no consciousness to rule you.

Mastering sense consciousness gratification is one of the spiritual puzzle pieces everyone will have to find on their pathway to enlightenment. As you begin to open to your true spiritual nature, you will forego compulsive dysfunction from the brain. Fulfillment from your spirit can bring a contentment that goes off the brain's scale to feel good, with the side effects being benefits.

Do The Practice and one day, addiction will become a distant memory, not a reality today.

Guilt is the soul's version
of quicksand.

Guilt is just another name
for a compartment in the
Kelee

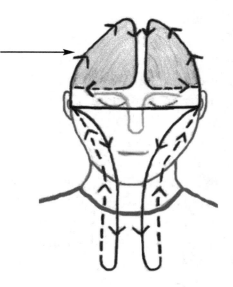

Letting go of guilt is one of the puzzle pieces everyone must master to be free.

Whenever you do something knowingly or out of a lack of awareness and it goes wrong, guilt can form. The way to deal with guilt is first by awareness of it, second by understanding that if you're feeling guilt, it has already compartmentalized in you. Detachment is the only recourse at this point.

Stepping into guilt is like stepping into quicksand, the more you struggle the deeper in you get. Remember, your mind always senses what's in front of you, if you're mindful. *Awareness is a powerful tool in your mind.* If you sense what will hurt you before you do something, you will not do it. It's better to do nothing than do something you knowingly will regret. When your mind knows what not to do, your brain does not have to think about it. Your spirit knows how to keep you out of trouble when a spiritual puzzle piece is in place to protect you.

When guilt has really gotten out of control, it can be used to control others. Have you ever had someone try to "guilt you?" When someone tries to control you by guilting you, try this: simply ignore what the person has said, as if they had said nothing at all and move on to something more worthwhile. It's a great technique and bewildering to dysfunction.

You can walk away from the guilt trips of others, but if you feel guilt in your own mind, you live with it. Remember, guilt is not you; it's only a compartment. Compartments looked at in the right way are signs pointing to puzzle pieces. You just need to learn how to read the signs.

*The minute
you stop judging another
is when you will be free from them.*

Civil law relates to your
outside world and your brain
i.e., intellect

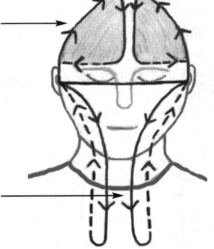

Spiritual law relates to your
inside world and your mind
i.e., spirit

There are two forms of judgment in the world: civil and spiritual. Civil laws are intellectual laws and need to be in place for people who have lost control of their mind. These people are high-maintenance humans. They cannot control themselves, so society has to. This form of judgment is necessary to maintain a sense of order in the world. When each individual takes responsibility for their malfunctioning compartments determining their actions, a judicial system one day will no longer be needed in the world.

The other form of judgment is spiritual in nature and has to do with how you perceive yourself or others. When you judge yourself harshly and unfairly, you have given yourself a sentence that no one can free you from. Who can get you out of this form of imprisonment? This is a version of hell.

If you judge another, you will not be free from them. When you judge someone, you carry around their problem in your mind. If you judge how another lives their life, it's as if you're saying, "You're not fit to run your mind, so I'll do it for you." Don't you have enough of your own problems to solve?

When you stop controlling, you will stop judging. Then you'll start having more time to find what non-judgment is really about—your freedom from your own mental imprisonment.

When you have to win
at any cost,
the cost is always too high.

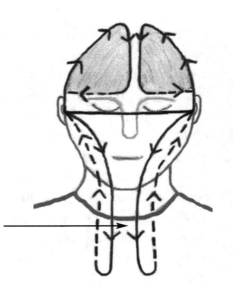

When your heart is in what
you do, you never lose

The brain by nature is competitive; it operates by the fight or flight response. The brain wants to be number one, but what if you're not? Are you worthless and do you beat yourself up? If you turn on yourself, you'll form depression. Now you not only feel like a loser, you're depressed too and you did it to yourself. Why?

Does what you do define who you are?

Being competitive and playing games challenges the mind and body, but never forget they're only games. If competition is not grounded in your spirit, you may try to win at all costs, with the price being too heavy. A wise man once said, "What profit a man to gain the whole world but lose his own soul?" To live by this philosophy is to be an eternal loser. When competition demeans others, no one wins. Win or lose, you can only be you. Remember, your life isn't ruined because you don't always win; it's ruined when you feel you have to.

The world is your playground, if you can learn to play in it. Everything in life, if it's any fun, is about play. How much fun do you have in your life?

Have you ever noticed, when you're looking for fun, you haven't found it. And when you're having fun, you don't have to look for it. When your heart's open to life, you start having fun.

*A need to get approval from others
is negating
your own approval of yourself.*

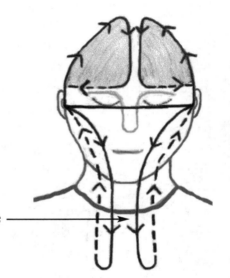

Approval is self-acceptance
realized by your spirit

People seek approval in two basic ways: for what they do and for who they are. When it comes to approval for what you do, you can only do your best and learn from the rest. If you're learning and growing, what more can be asked of you?

When it comes to approval for who you are, it's your birthright. What or whoever gave you the idea that you need acceptance from another anyway?

If you look closely at the need to get approval, it stems from your own insecurity. You doubt your own mind i.e., spirit. As you get rid of the compartments that make you feel inferior, you'll open to your spirit and your need for outside approval will disappear. The experience of life that brings self-acceptance cannot be felt through the intellect, only realized within your mind i.e., spirit.

Do The Practice and your own light heart and happy experience of life will become the ultimate approval. It's ironic, when you don't need approval is when you always have it.

When something is right, you need no approval. When something is wrong, no approval can be given.

The acceptance everyone is looking to find is their own. Everyone will need this understanding one day to be complete. When you truly accept the beauty of your spirit, you will realize that outside approval is not needed.

*True beauty
is how you see yourself,
not how someone else sees you.*

The brain understands
beauty by how you look

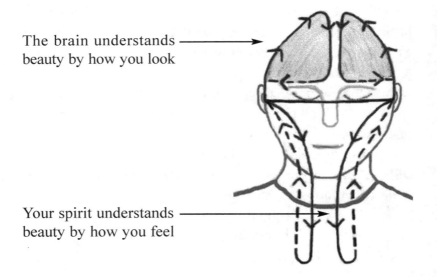

Your spirit understands
beauty by how you feel

The physical form of beauty will open any door, but how long you're welcome depends on inner beauty. Physical beauty is never hard to look at, but the absence of inner beauty can be.

You can perceive beauty from your head or from your heart. If physical beauty feeds your ego, your beauty has gone to your head and turns ugly. However, if you feel beautiful from your heart, it's always a warm contented feeling.

A beautiful spirit will always be a beautiful spirit, no matter what the outward appearance. If you're not feeling beautiful inside, you're missing a spiritual puzzle piece. How much would this puzzle piece be worth to you?

As you do The Practice your mind will brighten as the darkness of compartments disappear with the beauty of your spirit starting to shine. When your heart is truly happy, you glow. When you sense a glow coming from someone, it comes from the light of awareness. This light is also known as an aura, depicted in so many paintings of saints and sages. Your spirit has a beauty that never fades and only continues to grow deeper with the experience of time.

Your own spiritual beauty is a gem of understanding that makes you and the rest of the world a more beautiful place to be. Just imagine if everything you touched became more beautiful. It can happen.

If your heart feels beautiful, everything you touch becomes more beautiful. It is as simple as that.

Your self-image
is not what you see from your brain,
it's determined
by how you feel from your spirit.

Self-image is perceived
from your spiritual eyes
not your physical ones

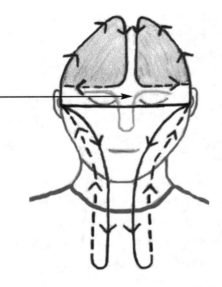

If you have to put on a good face, what does that say about the one behind it? Sadly, that you're unhappy with yourself. The problem is with how you see yourself. Problems with self-image are not changed by your outward appearance, but by how you see yourself from within through your spiritual eyes.

A negative self-image can manifest as: anorexia, bulimia, endless plastic surgeries and many other problems, all in an effort to try to change the way you feel about yourself. The brain tends to never be satisfied; there's always something better and more that can be done. The problem with the brain is, it sees from the outside in while your spirit sees from the inside out.

You're a dual being—physical and spiritual—and must master your physical body or you'll have problems. The problems invariably will be because of compartments showing you a negative image of yourself. When your conscious awareness can't see your self-image correctly, it's because of missing puzzle pieces in your spirit. If you cannot lovingly see your physical body with your spiritual eyes, you never will until the spiritual puzzle piece is found.

As you do The Practice and open to your spirit free from compartments altering your clear perception, you'll begin to see and experience yourself differently. You will see the magnificence of your physical self. Everyone is quite remarkable when viewed from their spirit.

If you do not see yourself as beautiful, you are not seeing the real you.

Culture
is the face of your soul,
but not the depth of your spirituality.

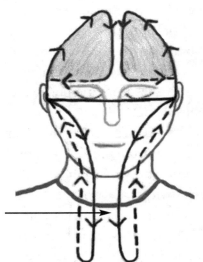

Your true nature is indigenous
to your own spirit

We are all indigenous to the earth somewhere. Culture is what you are born into, but if you cling to it, it separates you from your spirit. Many people in the world define themselves by their culture, but does culture define us or are we something deeper?

Your spirit does not have a culture, it's non-physical; it's not defined by how you look outside but how you are inside. Our physical presence exists only through viability. It takes your spirit to experience the understanding that a feeling of separation between people causes disharmony. The ultimate unity occurs within your own spirit, not from your culture.

Being indigenous with your spirit is one of the puzzle pieces associated with letting go of a need to have an outside identity. If you have to project an identity in front of you, who is the person projecting the persona? Why can't you just be yourself? Inevitably, this will be because you feel insecure with yourself, which invariably will come from a compartment that's not the real you.

What do you think will happen if you don't have a cultural self-image? Do you think you'll disappear as a person? It's all an elaborate mind game.

When you're native with your own spirit, you'll feel indigenous anywhere.

When you don't exclude yourself
from the world,
you become a part of it.

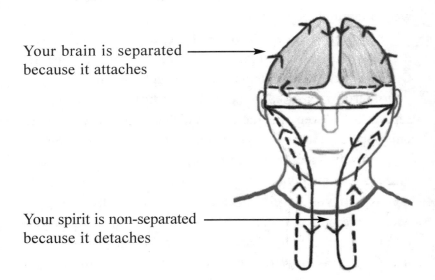

Your brain is separated
because it attaches

Your spirit is non-separated
because it detaches

The brain by physical nature is separated into two parts: the right and left hemispheres. If you live predominately in the brain, you end up feeling separated from the world. It's understandable why you may feel separated, the brain actually is!

The harder your brain tries to connect to the world, the more removed you feel from it. The brain is the physical part of you and attaches to the world, giving you an illusion of self-control. Your spirit is non-physical and detaches from the world, giving you the real form of self-control by not controlling at all.

Your spirit is without matter; it has never been separated by mass. The only separation your spirit will feel is from your missing spiritual puzzle pieces. When you live from your spirit it never closes you down, it opens you up to explore what you're missing.

Have you ever noticed if you think from your brain that your life is happy, you're still questioning it? However, when you're feeling happy from your heart, you don't need to check with your brain to see if you really are happy.

Happiness is the appreciation of being alive from your spirit open to the experience of life.

When you end the struggle of existence from your brain, and open to the absence of separation from your spirit, you'll find yourself at home anywhere. To understand the oneness of all things, you must feel the non-separation within your spirit.

*Expectations
are the prelude
to disappointment.*

Expectations are mental ⟶
attachments to an outcome

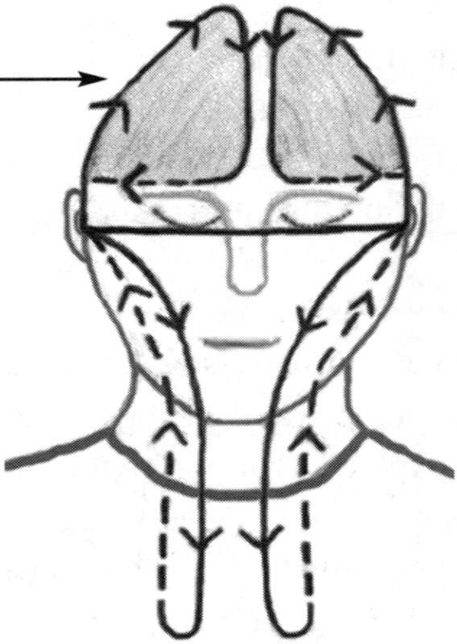

It's easy to have expectations about how things should be in the world, but changing how things are is a whole other thing! How often does the world do what you want? And if it doesn't act according to your dictates, whose problem is it?

The world is an unstable place; it's an absolute variable that will not sit still to please you. Having expectations about how the world should be is the breeding ground for headaches, if you cannot let go of your expectations. The only thing you can control in the outside world is what's in your own hands and that's temporary at best.

When you learn to detach through The Practice and dissolve compartments i.e., mental attachments, you will learn to let the world be. It's going to do what it's going to do anyway!

When you have expectations in your personal relationships, they can become painful heartaches. When your want is not fulfilled by another and your expectation is not fulfilled, your heart hurts. When out of fear, you attach to another, what you hold onto is what you must carry. If what you hold in your mind is an expectation of another that turns into dissatisfaction, your expectation will become a compartment. Once again, as you will hear many times, detachment is the answer. Expecting another to love you is taking away their ability to love you freely.

Feel your heart. If you truly love someone and can let them go, it's real love. Even if this someone walks away, don't you still love them?

Remember, not having an expectation of love is actually how you open to it.

Sexuality
when misunderstood
becomes a confused version of love.

Sex is associated with the brain ——→

Love is associated with the spirit ——→

In society, if we talk about a lover, it's someone we have sex with. Yet whether we truly love this person is more determined after the sexual act than before. Sexuality is only a temporary feeling from the lesser part of us. It's the highest of the low in us, at best.

Sexuality without puzzle piece understanding can be frustrating when run by sense consciousness cravings in the brain. Sexual feelings when not grounded in love are often followed by a feeling of emptiness that something is missing. If sexuality is not felt from a loving place in your spirit, you feel left out of the experience and feel a void. This void is from missing spiritual puzzle pieces associated with sexuality.

What everyone is really looking to find is the deeper eternal feeling found from realizing the missing puzzle pieces in your spirit. When it comes to sexuality, there are multiple spiritual puzzle pieces to find which are hard to describe in words. Let's just say, if you're having trouble feeling comfortable with sexual issues, you're missing a spiritual puzzle piece.

Invariably, along with missing puzzle pieces comes the baggage you pick up by mistake; this baggage is actually a pointer and a clue to what you're missing. As you do The Practice and the baggage dissolves, a clear space will appear in your spirit. Stand still in this clear place and ponder your problem. It's from this spiritual space of pondering that one day you will realize why you had the problem and how to free yourself from it.

When you're alone
with love,
you will never be lonely again.

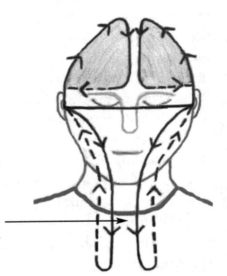

Mastering aloneness is the
center puzzle piece of your
spirit

When you cannot be alone, it's because your conscious awareness is not comfortable with your spirit. The alone puzzle piece is in fact the most important puzzle piece of your spirit. It is referred to by masters as, "The Bigee." If you do not have this puzzle piece, you're missing your center. If you fear being alone and do not like it at your deepest level, you fear your own spirit.

If you're alone and fear it, what do you think will happen? Nothing. The fear is all an illusion! Without understanding your own beautiful nature, this fear can torment you relentlessly.

It can be a very scary thing to look within your spirit. There seems to be this fear in humans that if you truly look at yourself, you might be ugly and no one will love you. The only thing ugly is your compartments and they're not the real you. The fear of being ugly can't be further from the truth. Your spirit is more beautiful than you can imagine.

If you can't be alone and feel love for yourself, you will never have a loving relationship. If you need to have others around to support you, your need will take energy from them. This need will make you a high-maintenance human because you can't sustain yourself from your own spirit.

If you're not open to your spirit, you'll never allow anyone close to you. You'll push away the very love you want, out of fear of getting hurt, ironically, while you're already hurting.

As you dissolve what isn't you—fear—you'll find what is the beauty of your true nature. Whenever you are by yourself, imprint this in your brain until you feel it in your heart: *your spirit is beautiful.*

When you're not trying
to give love
is when you always do.

When you live from your ⎯⎯⎯⎯⎯⎯⎯
head, you think love

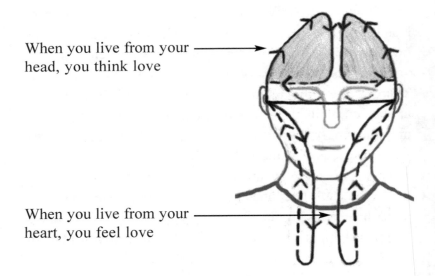

When you live from your ⎯⎯⎯⎯⎯⎯⎯
heart, you feel love

The giving and receiving of love is without a doubt the most difficult of all human experiences to work out. If you're afraid to feel your heart, you will not feel comfortable expressing love from it.

You cannot think your way into love. You must feel love directly yourself. The love you may think you need from others is actually the love you need to feel for yourself. The reason why you need is that you don't feel love in your own heart. The love you need to sustain yourself is not from your head but from your heart, open to your greater Kelee.

It is said, "It is better to give than to receive." However, if you don't feel love in your heart, giving doesn't happen, taking does. Giving from a need to get something in return is not giving, but a give to get and inevitably a painful experience. Love always gives itself and is never at the expense of anyone. When you're not trying to give, you give naturally; it's called being yourself.

The giving of love is understood by learning why you're closed off to love or why you're not open to love, or both. If you're closed to love, it's because of a painful compartment. If you're not open to love, it's because you don't know how to love because of a missing puzzle piece.

People struggle with love because they're afraid to feel out of fear. If you really want to feel love, you must risk opening your conscious awareness to your heart. Then you'll give to yourself that which is your birthright, your loving acceptance of who you really are—your spirit.

*When you're open
to your spirit,
you can receive from it.*

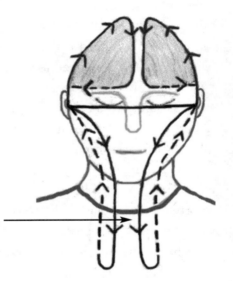

Your spirit opens when it's
not blocked by painful
compartments

When it comes to receiving love, it can be a scary experience. As the old saying goes, "It is better to give than to receive." However, isn't it a lot harder to receive? You must be vulnerable to receive.

When you drop your guard and stop protecting yourself, what comes at you first is your own pain. If pain is in between your conscious awareness and your spirit, how can you feel love? If your pain blocks your ability to receive love, you'll be forced to operate from your head with all of the expectations, attachments and strings associated with the intellect. When you detach from your pain and open to your heart, acceptance of love happens.

If you cannot receive, what can be given to you? The love you want to receive from another is actually the love you need to feel yourself. You receive love when you open your heart to love. When you have love in your heart, you don't need to get love from someone else, you already have it.

Love is not a linear measure from your head, it's an endlessly flowing fountain felt within your spirit. Do The Practice and you'll stop protecting yourself from the pain blocking you from the source of love. Remember, pain is the prelude to love, not love itself. Love never hurts, only the absence of love hurts.

The greatest treasure you will ever find is love and it's found by opening your heart. The map to your treasure is the greater Kelee. What you do with it is up to you.

*Compassion
is a flower that grows
from the soil of pain.*

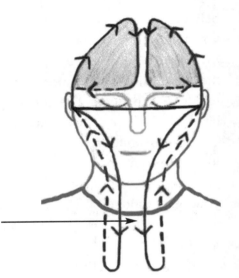

Compassion grows out of
the understanding of pain

Emotional pain is directed in two ways: against yourself or against others. If you have not faced your own pain, you will not want to feel another's. Their pain will mirror yours and if you don't want to look at it, you'll either inflict your pain on them or shut down yourself! Inflicting your disharmony on another is a perpetual pathway of suffering, commonly referred to as hell. You cannot live for long shutting down others or being shut down yourself, that's why you must master compassion.

To understand compassion, you must understand your own pain first. Let's face it, everyone would rather be doing something other than facing their inner torment or another's, but it's everywhere! Compassion cannot be intellectually manufactured from the head; that's pacification, an imitation of compassion. Compassion is realized from having felt deep pain and never forgotten it.

Compassion is attained when you cross the threshold of pain into the realization of knowing why suffering happens. Compassion is the healing aspect of love and will heal any of your soul's wounds. If you are to help another, you must have helped yourself first.

As you do The Practice and remove the rocks of pain from your soul, the flower of compassion will start to grow within you. When your suffering has blossomed into the flower of compassion, your loving presence becomes a precious gift to all you touch.

*The steps to enlightenment
cannot be understood
until you take them.*

Your intellect speculates by
thinking

Your spirit realizes by
feeling

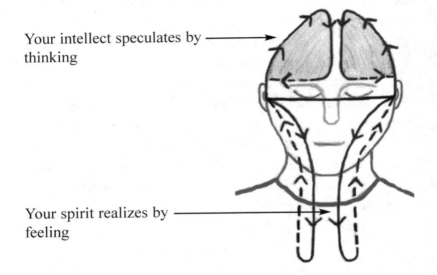

The robes of enlightenment do not look like anything that can be seen with the physical eyes because enlightenment is a spiritual process, not an intellectual one.

The distinguishing difference between an intellectual understanding of spirituality and realization from spiritual puzzle pieces is whether suffering remains or not. Enlightenment is the process by which we free ourselves from suffering; this can only happen if you really understand! You cannot understand enlightenment until after spiritual realization has happened. Speculation of enlightenment is theory.

Spiritual puzzle pieces are realized when your spirit understands something it has never understood before in your existence as an entity. When your conscious awareness is not being distracted by speculation from the intellect and not being blocked by compartments, you will open to your spirit to receive life uninterrupted. A previous problem is viewed like never before and a spiritual puzzle piece is born. This is the true meaning of being "born again." From that moment on you will never repeat the same mistake.

The path to finding all of your puzzle pieces is long, but the only thing that matters is, are you enjoying the walk? Don't worry about life; learn from it, it's what you're here to do.

You may not know right now where The Practice will take you, but doesn't it look all too real and a beautiful way to go?

Appreciation

As the founder of The Practice, I would like to express to everyone, that the knowledge of the Kelee is here for you. In reading this book you will gain the intellectual knowledge of the Kelee, but you will only understand what it really means when you do The Practice for an extended period of time.

Remember, The Practice is a way to help you find yourself. When you're in harmony, you will be an example of harmony. Everything you need to find your way is here, you just have to do The Practice and the beauty of your life will open in front of you.

As you learn, you will have experiences to share and what better way to share than that which touches your heart. The Kelee is a priceless treasure map to your heart and a way to find what is most important in life—love.

If your heart is touched by what you have received from this book and you would like to give back—feel free to do so. Your generosity and thankfulness will be most appreciated.

You may send your thank you to:

Ron Rathbun
P.O. Box 373
Oceanside, CA 92049-0373

About the Author

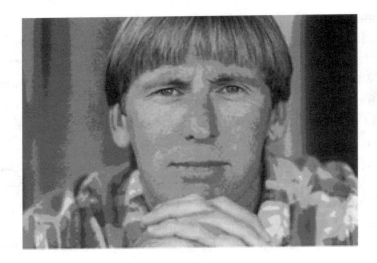

Ron Rathbun grew up in a middle class environment in what was then a small town. His early years were much the same as those of millions of people across America in the latter part of the twentieth century. Through some extraordinary events that happened early in his life, he was lead inward to ultimately find and explore the Kelee. Everyone who can feel knows the Kelee is real. You have felt emotions coming out of it your whole life.

Ron developed The Practice for himself, to free himself from his own pain so that he could open to the beauty of life. He feels that it's not so important that you know about him, it's more important that you know about yourself. If you want to understand your life, you must understand your own mind.

There are times in fortunate people's lives when they glimpse the eternal. What can be said when it happens to one at a young age and continues to evolve as a continuous stream of experience throughout one's life? The Kelee will help all to glimpse the eternal through The Practice.

Ron is the author of two other books. *The Way is Within* was compiled and written in his early years of study and teaching. It is very dear to his heart and the essence of who Ron is can be felt on its pages. As Ron continued to teach, students would ask him, "How did you connect to your true nature? How can I?" As a result, he wrote *The Silent Miracle*. It is a beautiful preview to *The Kelee*. *The Kelee* is Ron's gift for you. All you have to do to receive from it is to do The Practice.

Index

Index

Index

Index

The Kelee

Each copy of *The Kelee* is $25.00 plus shipping. Book description: Hardcover, 375 pages, 5.5 x 8.5. Please specify how many you wish to order.

Book Order: #_____@ $25.00 each   **Amount:** $ _____

Sales Tax: CA residents add applicable sales tax   _____

Shipping: Book Rate: $3.50 for the first book   _____

Add $1.00 for each additional book   _____

Surface shipping—allow 3 to 4 weeks

Air Mail: $5.00 per book   _____

Total: $ _____

Payment Method:

Check or money order payable to Quiescence Publishing in U.S. funds only

Mail Order To: Quiescence Publishing
P.O. Box 373
Oceanside, CA 92409-0373
760.439.1005

Ship To:

Name _____

Address _____

City _____ State _____ Zip _____

Telephone _____

How did you hear of *The Kelee*?
Please check out our website: www.ronrathbun.com
ISBN: 0-9643519-8-6